The Handbook of

BACH FLOWER REMEDIES

for Animals

of related interest

Passionate Medicine
Making the Transition from Conventional Medicine to Homeopathy
Edited by Robin Shohet
ISBN 978 1 84310 298 4

When a Family Pet Dies
A Guide to Dealing with Children's Loss
JoAnn Tuzeo-Jarolment, Ph.D.
Foreword by Linda Tintle
ISBN 978 1 84310 836 8

The Chinese Book of Animal Powers
Chungliang Al Huang
ISBN 978 1 84819 066 5

FOREWORD BY DR RICARDO OROZCO

ENRIC HOMEDES

TRANSLATED BY DANIEL KAI

The Handbook of

BACH
FLOWER
REMEDIES

for Animals

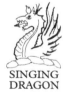

SINGING
DRAGON

LONDON AND PHILADELPHIA

Chapter 10 is reproduced with kind permission from the Altarriba Foundation, Spain.

This English translation published in 2011
by Singing Dragon
an imprint of Jessica Kingsley Publishers
116 Pentonville Road
London N1 9JB, UK
and
400 Market Street, Suite 400
Philadelphia, PA 19106, USA

www.singingdragon.com

First published in Spanish by Enric Homedes in 2009

Copyright © Enric Homedes 2009 and 2011
Translation copyright © Daniel Kai 2011
Foreword copyright © Dr Ricardo Orozco 2009 and 2011

Library of Congress Cataloging in Publication Data
Homedes, Enric.
[Manual de flores de Bach aplicadas a los animales. English]
The handbook of Bach flower remedies for animals / Enric Homedes ;
translated by Daniel Garc?a-Tapetado ; foreword by Ricardo Orozco.
   p. cm.
Includes bibliographical references and index.
ISBN 978-1-84819-075-7 (alk. paper)
1. Homeopathic veterinary medicine. 2. Alternative veterinary medicine. 3.
Flowers--Therapeutic use. 4. Homeopathy--Materia medica and therapeutics. I.
Title.
SF746H6613 2011
636.089'55--dc22
                            2011007705

British Library Cataloguing in Publication Data
A CIP catalogue record for this book is available from the British Library

ISBN 978 1 84819 075 7

Printed and bound in Great Britain

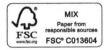

To Boby

Contents

5 Most Common Behavioural Problems 103

10 Neutering   237

FOREWORD

This book undoubtedly fills an important void in the Bach Flower literature. I am convinced it will henceforth be a link between Flower Remedies and our friends, the animals.

This is an honest and well-researched work. Those of us who know Enric Homedes are aware that he energetically defends and loves animals, which results in his daily work with and for them. This commitment involves the study of their temperament, psychology, instincts and their life in captivity. Furthermore, and this is no minor issue, I often see how, through our ignorance, we try to understand animal behaviour by projecting ourselves onto them, asking questions such as 'What would I do in their place?' It is easy to conclude that the result of this is confusion, which, as the author points out, results in many cases of abandoning or putting down the poor animal. 'Putting to sleep' seems to be a sweetened euphemism.

However, what I actually admire most in this book is that it is written by someone whose knowledge of the Bach Flowers dates back a long time and who has a great deal of experience with them.

I am very enthusiastic about the extensive case studies it contributes, demonstrating that it is not written as speculation from an indulgent and sedentary point of view, but as a product of methodical, and above all serious, constant practice. I find that many Flower Therapists, when we are faced with any Bach Flower sceptic, argue its quick effect on animals, babies and plants, where the placebo effect is obviously impossible.

Homedes' professional experience, described in part in this book, reminds us once again that Bach Flower Therapy is not a matter of faith, but of technical knowledge, good practice and method.

I hope this work is distributed as widely as it deserves and helps those wonderful beings that offer us everything in exchange for almost nothing: animals.

Dr Ricardo Orozco
Barcelona, February 2009

Acknowledgements

First of all, I would like to thank my wife, Carmen Roig, who has been an essential collaborator in my dedication to Flower Therapy and particularly in the preparation of this book. Without her collaboration this book would have been less meaningful, or maybe would not have even been possible.

The present acknowledgements must also include the valuable contribution of the following people and entities:

I would like to thank SEDIBAC (Society for the Study and Promotion of Bach Flower Remedies in Catalonia) and my fellow board members. Also my thanks go to the team of volunteers, as well as their coordinators, Josep Lluís Pujol and Carme Roig. I thank each and every one of them for the support, backing and appreciation they have always shown me. I am grateful to Teresa Coll for her help, encouragement and suggestions, and also for her conviction that this work would be completed.

I would like to thank Emily McClave, Lisa Clark and Jessica Kingsley Publishers/Singing Dragon, publishers of this book. I thank Daniel Kai for his translation into English, Susan Martin for the final review, and Pinnucia Strippol for her translation into Italian.

I would like to thank Neus and Luigi for lending me their house at Queralbs, where my work was made easier by the natural environment.

I would also like to express my gratitude to three important personalities of the Flower Therapy world: Lluís Juan Bautista,

Ricardo Orozco and Eduardo Grecco. They have been important cornerstones in developing and consolidating my career as a Bach Flower teacher and therapist.

My special thanks go to Jorge Quiroga, dog trainer and director of the dog training school Escuela de Educación y Formación Canina en positivo Single Track, and to the veterinarian Enric Infante, for their great help in the review of the present work and for their professionalism in their respective fields.

I would like to remember Barbara, Toni and the rest of the volunteers at the Amics dels Animals de la Noguera animal shelter who every day take care of the 180 dogs and cats in the shelter, in a totally altruistic manner, and under the harsh conditions of a country where the laws for animal protection are not complied with. Our work together and close collaboration has enabled us to extend our knowledge.

I am also grateful to Lidia and Josep María, volunteers at the animal shelter, for their kindness, hospitality and great affection showed from the moment we arrived there.

Of course I also thank my dear friends Encarna and Joan, *els boletaires* ('mushroom collectors'), for their great, unconditional love for animals.

Finally, my gratitude to the other organizations and foundations that promote the protection, welfare and adoption of abandoned animals, especially the Foundation for the Adoption, Sponsorship and Defence of Animals (FAADA), the Association for the Defence of Animal Rights (ADDA) and the Altarriba Foundation.

Enric Homedes

Introduction

Many cats and dogs have unnecessarily been put down when manifesting behavioural problems. Unlike humans, animals often do not have the opportunity to deal with their primary emotions such as fear, aggressiveness, anxiety, stress or depression.

After administering Bach Flower Remedies to animals for several years, I have found that animals respond quicker to treatment than humans. Animals experience emotions in a more straightforward way, without rationalizing them, without intellectual analysis and without the need to integrate or accept the emotion they experience. They feel and express emotions immediately, fully and intensely.

Bach Flower Remedies are increasingly being acknowledged by the veterinary world and canine trainers, and are being used to a greater extent by the professionals in these fields, especially in situations where animals need help to reduce their stress levels.

The main aim of the work outlined in this book, approached from a Flower Therapist's point of view, is to spread the application of Flower Remedies throughout the animal world in the occupations mentioned above, as well as among animal owners, and in animal shelters and the various organizations that promote the protection and adoption of abandoned animals.

The great benefit that Bach Flower Remedies offer for adopted animals should be emphasized, because they make the animal's adaptation to its new home easier, thus avoiding unnecessary 'returns'.

This is a practical handbook designed to help readers find solutions to the most frequent behavioural problems in the animal world, thereby improving animals' coexistence with and adaptation to the world around them (e.g. other animals, babies, children, their owners, the environment, etc.). However, it is not in any way intended that it should replace the work of the vet, canine trainer or behaviourist. When animals manifest a behavioural problem, the first step is to take them to the vet in order to rule out the possibility that any of the changes in their behaviour are rooted in a physical problem. In any therapy used to address behavioural problems, one must always consider how much of the responsibility for the animal's anomalous behaviour falls on the owner or the environment in which the animal lives. In this respect, the advice of an behaviourist or canine trainer must be considered essential, as they can teach the owners not to humanize their animal's feelings and to discern when its behaviour, although troublesome, is part of its intrinsic nature and when it is pathological.

Finally, I would like to stress the need for close collaboration between veterinary professionals, canine trainers and Flower Therapists to guarantee the correct solution to an animal's behavioural problem.

Who was Dr Edward Bach?

Edward Bach[1] was born in 1886 at Moseley, Birmingham (England). At the age of 20, after three years working in his father's brass foundry, he joined the Medicine School at Birmingham University, qualifying as a doctor in 1912 at London's Royal College of Surgeons. In 1915 he opened his private practice in London. Dr Bach studied disease by observing the way each patient reacted to a disease's characteristics (duration, severity, etc.). He concluded that the same remedy did not always cure the same disease in all patients and that, when treating a disease, the patient's personality was more important than the body.

He then became an Assistant Bacteriologist at University College Hospital, London. His work and research established a relationship between intestinal toxaemia and chronic disease. He noted that certain intestinal germs were directly related to chronic disease, and he prepared a vaccine based on those germs. Despite being very successful, he was not fully satisfied with his work because some diseases were not cured by the treatment and the patients still suffered the pain of the syringes.

During the First World War he was put in charge of 400 war beds at University College Hospital and was Clinical Assistant of Bacteriology. In 1917 he had a severe haemorrhage and lost consciousness for around 24 hours. The doctors gave him three months to live. He became obsessed with the idea that he had only

---

1   Based on the biography of Dr Bach by Nora Weeks (1940).

three months left to finish his research and worked day and night in his investigations. Some months later he recovered his health.

In 1919 he was accepted as Bacteriologist and Pathologist at the London Homeopathic Hospital. There he became inspired by and came to agree with the work of Samuel Hahnemann, who believed that a real cure meant curing the patient and not the disease, and that medication should be applied according to the patient's mental symptoms and not the physical ones. From that moment on, Dr Bach prepared vaccines using the homeopathic procedure. He then created the 'Seven Bach Nosodes', which were oral vaccines based on seven different intestinal bacteria isolated from chronically ill patients. He also noted that the Seven Nosodes corresponded to seven different human personality types, and therefore decided to treat his patients according to their emotional symptoms.

In 1928 he started to observe the people around him and noted that he could divide all of them into different personality groups. He would then monitor this in every patient that attended his practice. He was convinced that the definitive cures were to be found in plants and trees, and following his instinct he travelled to Wales where he collected three plants: Impatiens, Mimulus and Clematis. He was completely convinced that these plants could replace his bacterial nosodes.

Early in 1930 he set off again for Wales. He forgot all his laboratory equipment but soon found a new method of preparing the remedies which needed no sophisticated methodology. One day, early in the morning, he observed the dew resting on the plants and thought that this liquid could contain the properties and powers of each plant. He decided to carry out experiments by collecting flowers from different plants and placing them in bowls filled with water. He found out that the sun's light was essential and that it would enhance the plant's vibrations. In 1930 he perfected the 'sun method' and wrote his book *Heal Thyself* (Bach 1931). The book explains the principles of this way of healing and that the causes of disease are not essentially physical, but a consequence of moods and states of mind. It describes how the mind has control over the body and how the mind can heal the body.

Between 1930 and 1931, Bach found most of the 12 remedies he then called the 'Twelve Healers'. The 'Twelve Healers' correspond to 12 states of mind in the following categories: fear, uncertainty, insufficient interest in present circumstances, loneliness, over-sensitivity to influences and ideas, despondency or despair, and over-concern for the welfare of others. The 12 states of mind are: fear, terror, mental torture or worry, indecision, indifference or boredom, doubt or discouragement, over-concern, weakness, self-distrust, impatience, over-enthusiasm, and pride or aloofness.

In 1933 Bach completed the discovery of seven more remedies that he called the 'Seven Helpers', and in 1934 he published the second edition of the book *The Twelve Healers and the Seven Helpers* (Bach 1934).

Soon he would find the next 19 remedies, which would then complete his healing system. However, he discovered these last remedies in a totally different way: some days before he discovered a new remedy he would experience the same state of mind and suffering associated with that particular remedy. He completed his healing system with those 19 remedies in 1935. He died in his sleep on 27 November 1936.

1

HOW TO PREPARE FLOWER REMEDIES FOR AN ANIMAL

Preparation of a remedy for oral application (second dilution)

In a 60 ml (2 fl oz) amber-coloured glass dropper bottle, add mineral spring water and 4 drops of each of the selected remedies (plus 8 drops of Rescue Remedy if used). The Flower Remedies can be bought separately in 10, 20 and 30 ml (⅓, ⅔ and 1 fl oz) bottles, called stock bottles (first dilution or full strength), or in a full set containing the 38 Bach Flower Remedies and the Rescue Remedy. If a 30 ml (1 fl oz) dropper bottle is used, only 2 drops will be added of each remedy from the stock bottle (first dilution) and 4 drops of the Rescue Remedy if used.

Preservatives such as cognac or apple vinegar should not be used in preparations for animals, as many animals, particularly cats, will then reject the remedy combination. In times of intense heat the remedy combination can be conserved in the fridge.[1] A plastic bottle can substitute the glass dropper bottle, especially for

---

1   In some Flower Remedy workshops and conferences, I have heard that the remedy combination can be altered by the electromagnetic fields that fridges generate. Fortunately, all remedy combinations and eye-drops that we have stored in the fridges of animal shelters have continued to work when applied to animals. Animals and babies help us validate the efficacy of the Flower Remedies as they are placebo exempt.

very nervous or aggressive animals, as they could bite the pipette and hurt themselves.

It is advised that no more than seven remedies of the stock bottle set (first dilution) are selected to prepare the individual remedy formula. Using more remedies would cause the animal's system to be overwhelmed by the amount of 'information' in the formula, and so it would not be as effective. However, this book does describe some formulas that use more than seven remedies because several different aspects of the animal's condition were all considered a priority at the time.

Preparation of a remedy for local application

In the chapter on dosage methods included in *The Twelve Healers and Other Remedies* (Bach 1936), Bach himself described treatment using local application with the remedies he had discovered.

I quote various paragraphs from that book:

> *In those unconscious, moisten the lips frequently.*

> *Whenever there is pain, stiffness, inflammation, or any local trouble, in addition a lotion should be applied. Take a few drops from the medicine bottle in a bowl of water and in this soak a piece of cloth and cover the affected part; this can be kept moist from time to time, as necessary.*

> *Sponging or bathing in water with a few drops of the remedies added may at times be useful.*

After Dr Bach's death, the Rescue Remedy cream was commercialized; Rescue Cream contains the same remedies as the Rescue Remedy plus Crab Apple. Its application is recommended when there is a superficial trauma, burn, insect sting, sore, ulcer, psoriasis, infection, etc. This cream has proven effective in all those localized emergency situations with a topical manifestation.

At present, different practitioners have continued to work on treatments using local application of the Flower Remedies. Their experiences in the topical use of the remedies are gathered in several books. It is worth mentioning the work of Ricardo Orozco in his book, *Flores de Bach: Manual de Aplicaciones Locales* (*Bach Flowers: Handbook of Local Applications*) (Orozco 2003), where the concept of 'Patrón Transpersonal' (Transpersonal Pattern) is referred to. The author defines it as: 'the flower applications that do not come prescribed according to characteristics of personality. The interpretation does not focus on why something happens, but on the way in which it manifests itself, translating this manifestation into the Flower language' (p.25).

The concept of 'Transpersonal Pattern' is applied in the preparation of creams, eye-drops, sprays, compresses, massage oils, etc. For example, Vervain is used for idealist people who become inflamed when faced with any kind of injustice. By establishing a Transpersonal Pattern of inflammation for Vervain, Orozco thereby recommends the remedy for any problem that involves inflammation. The Transpersonal Pattern does not, however, treat the cause of the symptom. It deals only with manifestations of the conflict (sometimes expressed physically), as interpreted through Floral language.

Preparation of a Flower cream

Use a neutral cream base to prepare creams. In areas with necrosis or which show more redness after applying the cream, substitute the cream base with a 99 per cent Aloe Vera gel (acting as a cellular regenerator).

Containers of different measurements are available on the market. The most usual ones are 10 ml (⅓ fl oz), 30 ml (1 fl oz), 50 ml (2 fl oz), 100 ml (3½ fl oz), 150 ml (5 fl oz), 500 ml (18 fl oz) and 1000 ml (1¾ pints), which can be made of either glass or plastic. Before selecting the volume of the container, bear in mind the volume of cream necessary for each application. The treatment of an eyelid will not be the same as the treatment of a whole limb. I recommend buying a 1 kg (2¼ lb) jar of cream base and distributing it into containers with different volumes, using a wooden or plastic spoon or spatula.

To prepare a Flower cream, add 1 drop of each selected remedy of the stock bottles (first dilution) for every 10 ml (⅓ fl oz) of cream (2 drops of Rescue Remedy if used). For example, add 3 drops of each of the chosen remedies for a 30 ml (1 fl oz) container, 5 drops for a 50 ml (2 fl oz) container, and so on. For 50–100 ml (2–3½ fl oz) containers, 7 drops of each remedy will be enough, and from 500 ml (18 fl oz) upwards, do not add more than 10 drops of each of the selected remedies.

The number of chosen remedies for each container should not exceed seven. No preservative should be added, as each cream base manufacturer uses its own preservative.

Add the drops of each chosen remedy to the central part of the container and immediately stir clockwise with a wooden or plastic spatula until the drops are totally absorbed.

Application

The frequency of the application of a Flower cream depends on the case to be treated. Generally, two applications per day are enough, because this frequency normally seems to transmit sufficient energy information to be effective. However, in acute cases, quicker results have been achieved by applying the cream four times per day.

Preparation of Flower eye-drops

Sterile saline solution is the diluent vehicle used for the formulation of eye-drops. You should not add any preservative as the eye is a very sensitive organ.

Separate the three components of a 10 ml/⅓ fl oz dropper bottle (or one not larger than 30 ml/1 fl oz), that is, the bottle, glass dropper and plastic screw-on cap, and sterilize them by boiling them in water for ten minutes, in a stainless steel pot. After they have cooled down assemble the dropper bottle and add

10 ml of saline solution (chemists sell 5 and 10 ml monodoses) and a drop of each of the selected remedies from the stock bottle (first dilution).

APPLICATION

Apply 2 drops in each eye, a minimum of four times per day. If the eye-drop application is difficult, a sterile gauze can be impregnated with the prepared eye-drops and applied over the closed eyelid for a few moments. The external eye area must then be cleaned with the same gauze, especially if there is infection in the eye area.

2

ADMINISTERING THE FLOWER REMEDIES TO ANIMALS

Direct and Indirect Application, and How to Prepare Concentrate Formulas

Direct application

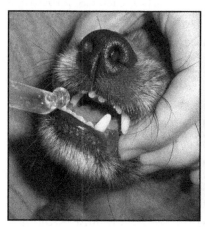 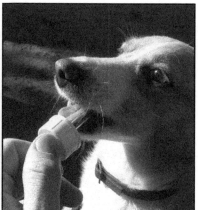

Direct application is the most common and effective form of oral application. Squeeze the equivalent of 4 drops from the amber-coloured bottle directly into the animal's mouth. Then clean the dropper with water by rinsing it under the tap, as saliva could generate a microorganism culture and contaminate the remedy combination. In the case of very fearful animals, those who present a certain type of aggressiveness or those who display stress when administering the Bach Flower Remedies (as is the case with some cats), the 4 drops can be squeezed onto their 'pet delicacy', favourite titbit or any porous food. Occasionally, we have poured the 4 drops onto a piece of bread with a bit of olive oil.

Another method of direct application is to use a needleless syringe to take in the equivalent of 4 drops of the personalized combination and administer it directly into the animal's mouth, usually through the side of the mouth, in the interdental space situated between the canine and the first premolar. This application is useful when you want to simultaneously treat animals living together in the same house with the same problems, or in a shelter, or in the case of some very nervous cats. The needleless syringe does not need to be refilled for each application and is quicker and safer to use than glass if cats react badly. Remember that plastic dropper bottles can also be purchased.

The daily number of doses will depend on each case. The usual way is to administer 4 drops four times a day. It is advisable to administer 4 drops six to eight times per day to animals that have been mistreated (for example greyhounds or former hunting dogs that have been adopted or are in shelters or temporary homes awaiting their adoption). In cases of serious mistreatment and torture, the duration of the treatment must not be less than six months.

There may be situations where administering the four minimum doses, spread out throughout the day, would be complicated for the owner. In these cases, we recommend combining direct application with indirect application, or that the owner administers the first dose on waking up, the second before leaving for work, the third on returning home, and the fourth before going to bed. It is better that the animal receives all four daily doses, even if the intervals between them are not equal, than it is to eliminate any of them.

Indirect application

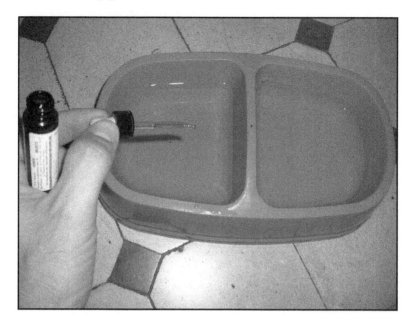

For several years my working procedure involved adding 15 to 20 drops of the personalized remedy combination to the water dish where the animal usually drinks. Despite seeing some encouraging results, I have found that indirect application is less effective than direct application. One hypothesis that would explain indirect application being less effective is the dilution effect. I therefore only recommend this method when the water dish the animal usually drinks from doesn't exceed 200 ml (7 fl oz).

In order to avoid the treatment being less effective when the only possible method is indirect application, I have found that it is more effective to add 5 to 15 drops[1] of each of the selected remedies from the bottles in the stock remedy set (first dilution) to the animal's water dish.

---

1 This will depend on the volume of the water dish each animal drinks from. Generally, 5 drops are enough in containers of 0.5 litres (18 fl oz) or less, 8 drops for 0.5 to 3 litre (18 fl oz to 5 pints) containers, and 15 drops for containers up to 10 litres (17½ pints). For bigger volumes, 25 drops will be enough.

Concentrate formula

When a Flower treatment needs to be administered to a large group of animals (in shelters, farms, zoos, etc.) which share a common pathology or behaviour, the formula is prepared in a different way. This formula will be called concentrate formula.

To prepare this formula, add 10 drops of each of the selected remedies to a 60 ml (2 fl oz) amber-coloured glass dropper bottle and fill the rest of the bottle with cognac. From this new formula, add 2 drops per litre of water in the animals' trough, up to a maximum of 25 drops.

3

RESCUE REMEDY

This formula consists of five of the 38 Flower Remedies that compose the Bach Flower system. They act together in synergy when an acute emergency situation arises. The five remedies are:

- Rock Rose for terror and panic

- Cherry Plum for fear of losing control, excessive rage and hysteria

- Impatiens for agitation, irritability and restlessness

- Clematis for weakness and self-absorption

- Star of Bethlehem for the relief of the effects of a shock.

This formula calms the animal in specific stressful situations, such as visits to the vet, preoperation procedures, a change of home, stress and panic reactions to fireworks, air travel, etc. (see Chapter 9). Consider this remedy for a psychological pregnancy or when an animal is in heat and very restless.

I must emphasize that the Rescue Remedy is not a base treatment; it does not treat the animal's character, but only stabilizes it during a specific stressful situation. Therefore, it will also be necessary to administer the remedies that deal with its character and those that tackle the behavioural patterns that might have generated or could generate a behavioural problem.

I have treated a lot of animals that showed clear signs of stress and panic after being found abandoned on highways or injured in car accidents, or showing clear signs of having been mistreated or poisoned. In most cases, I have found that these animals respond quicker to the treatment by giving them Rock Rose (panic) + Star of Bethlehem (shock), in addition to administering Rescue Remedy, despite the fact that those two remedies are both components of the Rescue formula. I have also found that if Sweet Chestnut (extreme anguish) is added together with the two aforementioned remedies, the results are even more positive. In cases of utmost urgency, that is, of very acute stress and panic, I also recommend adding Rescue Remedy to the formula composed of Rock Rose, Star of Bethlehem and Sweet Chestnut. This last flower manages extreme suffering and anguish, typical of an extremely stressful situation.

I would like to emphasize that I have no doubt whatsoever that the Rescue Remedy is effective; furthermore, if when treating any animal I only had Rescue Remedy available and not the remedies that compose it, I would administer the formula as it obviously carries out its purpose, that is as a stabilizing formula for a specific emergency moment. However, when you want to treat one or two emotions that are integrated in the Rescue Remedy formula, it is advisable to add them separately to the personalized remedy combination instead of using the Rescue Remedy.

4

STUDY OF EACH
OF THE 38 BACH
FLOWERS

In this chapter, the oral and local applications of the 38 Bach Flowers both for humans and for animals will be detailed. It has often been claimed that it is necessary to treat the animal and its owner simultaneously. This facilitates the action of the remedies administered to the animal and complements the recommendations of a canine trainer or behaviourist.

The study of each Flower Remedy opens with a quote by Dr Bach himself. Following the quote are descriptions of situations in the animal world where the efficacy of the flower has been proved, both orally and locally. The study closes with a description of the positive and negative qualities attributed to a person who manifests the personality or the state of mind that corresponds to the flower in question.

In the 'Application to animals' sections, following the names of the majority of the flowers, a word or short phrase in brackets (Key words) helps in understanding the reason for using that particular flower in the specific situation which is being described. Also in brackets, the sources from which the key word has been extracted are indicated with initials: E.B. (Bach 1936), TP (Orozco's (2003) Transpersonal Pattern), R.O. (Ricardo Orozco, physician, Flower Therapist and teacher; Orozco 2003), or P.N. (Pablo Noriega, expert in Traditional Chinese Medicine, acupuncturist and Flower Therapist; Noriega 2006).

This chapter is a practical guide to the most frequent uses of the Flower Remedies and is aimed at therapists trained in Flower Therapy, canine trainers, behaviourists, vets, people working with animals in rescue shelters and generally any person who loves animals.

4.1 Agrimony (Agrimonia eupatoria)

The jovial, cheerful, humorous people who love peace and are distressed by argument or quarrel, to avoid which they will agree to give up much.

Though generally they have troubles and are tormented and restless and worried in mind or in body, they hide their cares behind their humour and jesting and are considered very good friends to know. They often take alcohol or drugs in excess, to stimulate themselves and help themselves bear their trials with cheerfulness. (Bach 1936)

Application to animals

KEY WORDS: Anxiety (E.B.).

ORAL APPLICATION

Agrimony (anxiety) is the remedy suitable for the restless animal, which moves constantly from side to side and is never comfortable anywhere, and also for the stressed animal that lives in very limited spaces: shelters, rooms, cages with many dogs, etc. This remedy helps regulate anxiety and hyperactivity levels in animals in general.

Agrimony is part of the formulas that treat separation anxiety (refer to Section 5.2, p.111), coprophagia (refer to Section 5.4, p.115), stereotypic behaviour (refer to Section 5.7, p.120), and the behavioural problem of a dog eating everything it finds in the street.

Local application

As a cream or Aloe Vera gel, Agrimony is used for insect or other parasite bites and skin allergies of diverse nature (refer to Chapter 9, p.235).

Application to humans

Key words: Anxiety. Restlessness. Mental torment hidden under cheerfulness.

Agrimony people are permanently fleeing from themselves, fearing their own set of interior problems. In order to avoid coming into contact with their 'shadow', they need to be constantly moving and stimulated. They are very sociable people who present themselves to society with a mask of happiness and optimism, seeming to be unaffected by everything that happens around them. Agrimony people are 'party animals' and cannot stand silence or being inactive. However, their joy for life masks a deep anxiety and an extreme mental torment that often triggers some type of addiction, thus showing their tendency towards loss of control.

What underlies this is the need to be liked by others, which is why it is hard for the Agrimony person to say no, and why he or she will try to avoid any type of conflict.

Agrimony people normally minimize their problems. For them everything is perfect, wonderful and marvellous, and at the same time they do not face the negative and problematic aspects of their lives. Agrimony people hide their great interior torment, their lack of peace, serenity and calmness and their great anxiety, like a clown who laughs on the outside and cries on the inside.

Deep inside they are extremely sensitive, vulnerable and in need of harmony.

4.2 Aspen (Populous tremula)

Vague unknown fears, for which there can be given no explanation, no reason.

Yet the patient may be terrified of something terrible going to happen, he knows not what. These vague unexplainable fears may haunt by night or day.

Sufferers are often afraid to tell their trouble to others. (Bach 1936)

Application to animals

KEY WORDS: Disturbing fear.

ORAL APPLICATION

Aspen deals with disturbing fear and is used to treat animals that are very sensitive in nature and become restless with noises, movement of tree branches, breezes, etc.

Cats and horses are the animals that are most prone to fall under an Aspen state. This is because of their sensitivity and proneness to 'pick up' all types of presences and noises.

LOCAL APPLICATION

No known application.

Application to humans

KEY WORDS: Fear and anguish of unknown origin.

This type of fear is more like anguish. Some people, such as Dr Bach, describe it as panic, as can be appreciated from the quote above.

Aspen is useful for treating people who suffer sudden fears without any specific reason. They are nervous because they fear death or catastrophes. Those who suffer may be terrified or anguished when they have the intuition that something bad is going to happen without knowing exact details. These fears may occur suddenly when they are alone or in friends' company, and they may be afraid to confide their fears to others.

On many occasions, Mimulus is administered when the person can specify the type of fear he or she is experiencing, for example a fear of poverty, disease, death, darkness, cataclysms, etc. However, these fears are sometimes solved more quickly by taking Aspen when the person, although able to put a name to these fears, is in reality unaware of their origin and cause. Moreover, they have a feeling, almost a premonition, that whatever they do, something inevitable is going to happen.

4.3 Beech (Fagus sylvatica)

For those who feel the need to see more good and beauty in all that surrounds them. And, although much appears to be wrong, to have the ability to see the good growing within. So as to be able to be more tolerant, lenient and understanding of the different way each individual and all things are working to their own final perfection. (Bach 1936)

Application to animals

KEY WORDS: Intolerance (E.B. and TP). Irritability (E.B.). Irritation (TP). Rejection (TP).

ORAL APPLICATION

Beech (irritability) is one of the components of the aggressiveness formula (see Section 5.1, p.105). This remedy helps manage an animal's intolerance and rejection of another animal or a human.

It is of great help in those allergic processes and diseases that manifest as an irritative cough, such as kennel cough (see 'Kennel cough', p.225).

Beech is the remedy that treats the character type of many cats. It is part of the formula that treats lack of feline socialization (see Section 5.13.2, p.134). Cats find it difficult to tolerate changes, often urinating on the owners' clothes or bed in order to manifest their dissatisfaction when a new situation arises (see 'Defecation and urination in inappropriate places', p.118).

LOCAL APPLICATION

As a cream or Aloe Vera gel, Beech is useful for treating skin eczemas of an allergic nature, bites from insects or other parasites, hives and skin irritations in general. Beech is part of the formula used to treat mastitis.

It is applied as eye-drops in allergic and/or infectious conjunctivitis that manifests as irritation and also in the inflammation of the third eyelid (see Chapter 9).

Application to humans

KEY WORDS: Intolerance. Criticism.

Beech is the basic remedy that deals with intolerance. People in this state often seek errors and defects in others, and it is difficult for a Beech-type person to see the positive side of a person or situation. These characteristics frequently lead them to criticize and correct people around them, and they are easily made to feel irritated and indignant by others' defects and habits. They complain about unimportant situations and are rigid, strict and inflexible with anybody doing things differently from them. They also seek and demand perfection in everything that surrounds them, capable of arriving at a tyranny of aesthetics and perfection. Moreover, they are demanding and intolerant of the actions of others, while on the contrary being too indulgent and tolerant with themselves.

When unbalanced, they are arrogant, distant, cold, derogatory, proud and haughty. They do not tolerate superficiality or slackness, and they like orderliness on their own terms. They do not tolerate things being carried out badly because of lack of attention. Seeing a painting in a tilted position irritates them, not only for aesthetic reasons, but also because they are incapable of understanding the lack of attention to detail of the person responsible for hanging it.

Their arrogance sometimes gives you the impression that they are 'letting you off the hook'.

4.4 Centaury (Centarium umbellatum)

Kind, quiet, gentle people who are over-anxious to serve others. They overtax their strength in their endeavours.

Their wish so grows upon them that they become more servants than willing helpers. Their good nature leads them to do more than their own share of work, and in so doing they may neglect their own particular mission in life. (Bach 1936)

Application to animals

KEY WORDS: Weakness (TP). Submissiveness (E.B.).

ORAL APPLICATION

There are people who adopt or foster a dog in order to solve their own lack of affection, making the animal completely dependent on them. As time goes by this over-reliance on the owner can become a behavioural problem in the animal. One of the most common problems is separation anxiety (see Section 5.2, p.111). Centaury (submissiveness) is one of the remedies included in the separation anxiety formula.

There are animals that are submissive with people but dominant with other animals. In this case we have to consider what factors underlie this attitude and administer the remedies accordingly.

Centaury (weakness) is also a remedy that provides energy for both animals and humans. In some cases it can replace Olive (exhaustion) and in others strengthen its action. Both remedies are part of the formula that treats colds in animals (see Chapter 9, p.231).

This remedy is one of the components of the kennel cough formula (see p.227) and also of the formula that helps in the treatment of Leishmaniasis (see Case 6.8, p.166).

Local application

As a cream or Aloe Vera gel, and together with other remedies, Centaury has been used to treat ulcers and other dermatological problems (alopecia and desquamation) in animals suffering from Leishmaniasis. This remedy deals with a pattern of weakness and provides energy to weakened skin areas. Centaury has been chosen to treat this pathology because it is a disease of infectious aetiology and the animal must overcome the submission imposed by the characteristics of the disease itself (see Case 7.6, p.202).

Application to humans

KEY WORDS: Weak willpower and submissiveness.

Centaury's personality is of a passive, dependent nature that tends towards submissiveness. A Centaury person's kindness and altruism are greatly appreciated by other people. However, what really lies behind these two characteristics is Centaury's desire to be appreciated and loved, or in some cases the desire for protection by stronger personalities.

Not everybody needing this Flower Remedy has arrived to a Centaury state by being tyrannized against their will (as in Cinderella). Some are submissive to others because they seek protection. Others seek to merge and identify themselves with a person of a stronger nature. Centaury people have difficulty in decision-making and what they are really looking for is someone to take responsibility for every aspect of their life, including very basic everyday issues. Others have become Centaury because they have overprotective parents. They have imprinted an absolute dependence on them, creating a lack of self-confidence and low self-esteem, preventing them from starting their own projects or initiatives.

Some Centaury people were not born with that character type, but developed it because of their failure to win a power struggle with someone stronger (Beech, Chicory, Vervain, Vine). They became submissive and developed appeasement behaviours in order to ensure that they would not be destroyed by the stronger personality. They yielded, and continue to do so, in order to avoid violence by the stronger person to whom they are bound.

In Centaury there is a significant pattern of physical fatigue. Centaury people become exhausted because they give more than what they have, because they work excessively in order to please others and because they demand too much of themselves.

4.5 Cerato (Ceratostisgma willmottiana)

Those who have not sufficient confidence in themselves to make their own decisions.

They constantly seek advice from others, and are often misguided. (Bach 1936)

Application to animals

Key words: Confidence and sense of security (E.B.). Dispersion (TP).

Oral application

Cerato (dispersion) reinforces learning mechanisms, focusing the animal's attention on the guidelines to be learned. As in the case of Chestnut Bud (learning process) this remedy is suitable for animals attending training activities and being prepared for competitions and shows.

Local application
No known application.

Application to humans

Key words: Seeking advice and approval.

The people in need of this Flower Remedy may be intuitive but nonetheless constantly seek advice and approval from others. Their actions are always based on the last piece of advice they have received. They know what to do from the very beginning but need approval before taking action.

Cerato people can be mentally insecure, immature, irresponsible and indecisive. Cerato people always doubt everything and therefore cannot make decisions. They probably hesitate in order to avoid decisions and the consequent commitment to a specific action. They have difficulty distinguishing between right and wrong, between what is important and what is superficial. They normally lose track of what is essential.

Cerato people do not commit totally and are inconsistent. During the consultation they can be recognized by their need to ask many questions and their tendency to try to give up different treatments easily. At an intellectual level, they may be reading several books at the same time without finishing any one of them. They attend courses, conferences or seminars to accumulate the maximum amount of knowledge, although they normally do not put it into practice.

4.6 Cherry Plum (Prunus cerasifera)

Fear of the mind being over-strained, of reason giving way, of doing fearful and dreaded things, not wished and known wrong, yet there comes the thought and impulse to do them. (Bach 1936)

Application to animals

KEY WORDS: Lack of control (TP). Hysteria (E.B.).

ORAL APPLICATION

Cherry Plum (lack of control, hysteria) is one of the components of the aggressiveness formulas (see Section 5.1, p.105).

This remedy helps the dog that has gone crazy, victim of its own rage and hysteria. The remedy also treats the animal that shows an obsession with attacking other animals, and calms down its excited and obsessive mind. It is also suitable for the animal that is stressed due to living in a very limited space and is therefore unable to run around to release its excess energy (see Section 5.8, p.121).

Cherry Plum is used to treat animals that, although apparently calm and affectionate, suddenly attack without reason. It is important to ascertain whether a fear or trauma lie behind this behaviour (treatable with Rock Rose and Star of Bethlehem), or if there are states of Chicory (possessiveness over space, owner, objects, etc.), Heather (seeking attention), Vine (domination) or Holly (jealousy).

In some animals with Cherry Plum behaviour we must evaluate whether their aggressiveness is a result of antisocial behaviour. It is possible for this type of behaviour to arise in dogs that are taken away prematurely from their mothers when they were puppies and therefore did not experience a proper learning process; mothers are responsible for transferring important codes to them in their socialization process (a minimum period of four months). Cherry Plum behaviour may also show up in the cases of animals that were born with no genetic selection criteria when crossed (with the only purpose of the cross being to obtain more aesthetic and therefore more marketable breeds). In both cases, those animals may lack certain behaviour codes in adulthood, for example knowledge of what a human, a child, or a car is. Others may not be able to manage loud noises with relative calmness and some may get nervous if somebody wears an item of clothing (e.g. a hat or scarf) that they don't recognize or when smelling a person of a race unfamiliar to them. In either case it is recommended that Chestnut Bud be added to their formula. Chestnut Bud facilitates the animal's learning process for new situations and helps assimilate the guidelines that the canine trainer transmits in order to solve the Cherry Plum behaviour.

Cherry Plum is included in the formula that treats animals that suffer travel sickness and is a part of the kennel cough formula (see p.227).

Local application

No known application.

Application to humans

> **Key words**: Fear of going out of one's mind and losing control.

This remedy is appropriate for those who fear losing control or fear going crazy and are scared of doing something terrible against their own will. A person in a Cherry Plum state can have a sudden excess of rage and even suicidal thoughts.

The person in a Cherry Plum temperament represses all impulses that originate in the subconscious, accumulating tremendous internal pressure. This forces the repressed experiences to surface into consciousness and, when confronted with an external stimulus, provokes an explosion of hysteria and loss of control that leads to violent impulses that are directed towards themselves or others.

Cherry Plum not only helps patients who are overcome by the fear of losing control but also those who are already experiencing temporary madness and loss of control. It is also one of the five components of the Rescue Remedy.

4.7 Chestnut Bud (Aesculus hippocastanum)

For those who do not take full advantage of observation and experience, and who take a longer time than others to learn the lessons of daily life.

Whereas one experience would be enough for some, such people find it necessary to have more, sometimes several, before the lesson is learnt.

Therefore, to their regret, they find themselves having to make the same error on different occasions when once would have been enough, or observation of others could have spared them even that one fault. (Bach 1936)

Application to animals

KEY WORDS: Learning process (E.B.). Assimilation (TP).

ORAL APPLICATION

Chestnut Bud (learning process) is an indispensable tool for the canine trainer, the behaviourist and the Bach Flower Therapist as it allows the animal to learn behavioural guidelines more quickly. At the same time it helps the animal to assimilate the information received from the rest of the remedies in the Flower formula. This is why it is present in most Flower Remedy combinations that are intended to help the animal change behavioural patterns or inappropriate habits.[1] It is also used as the main remedy for animals with a lack of imprinting and socialization.

Chestnut Bud must be included in the formula to treat an animal that has difficulty adapting to a change: a house move, arriving at a new home (as a result of adoption, purchase, foster care, or being taken to an animal shelter), the arrival of a new

---

1   In some cases we have treated, we have reinforced the learning period with Clematis (facilitates attention), Cerato (trust and self-confidence) and Larch (disability).

animal or a baby, etc. It is also one of the components of the formula for treating feline social aggressiveness (see Section 5.1.5, p.110).

LOCAL APPLICATION

No known application.

Application to humans

KEY WORDS: Incapable of learning from past mistakes.

People in a Chestnut Bud state are naive, clumsy and misguided in their questions, bodily movements and actions. They often drop objects, trip over or spill food. They are hasty and reckless, and live the present moment quickly without paying much attention. They also have a tendency to escape from all that is unpleasant and uninteresting. Chestnut Bud people cannot assimilate the details of everyday life because they lack a good memory and the power of observation. They are superficial and immature. Moreover, they move from one situation to another without processing or assimilating them. Therefore, instead of learning from experience, they repeat the same mistakes over and over again.

Chestnut Bud children and teenagers always seem a bit distracted and inattentive. They do not register many things and have problems with concentration, memory and attention, resulting in learning problems.

4.8 Chicory (Cichorium intybus)

Those who are very mindful of the needs of others; they tend to be over-full of care for children, relatives, friends, always finding something that should be put right. They are continually correcting what they consider wrong, and enjoy doing so. They desire that those for whom they care should be near them. (Bach 1936)

Application to animals

KEY WORDS: Congestion (TP). Possessiveness (E.B.).
Retention (TP).

ORAL APPLICATION

Chicory (possessiveness) is the main remedy used to treat animals showing excessive territoriality and protectiveness towards their owner, other members of the family or objects. Usually the animal shows signs of aggressiveness when people or animals try to approach the territory, owner, family member, object or food in question (in the case of objects or food it would be considered protection of resources). What underlies this type of aggressiveness is a possessive character that tries to protect everything it believes is its own.

Some animals sense their owner's fear (fear for themselves, fear of their dog being attacked, fear of going out for walks at night, etc.) and interpret it as a sign of danger. They therefore manifest signs of aggressiveness in order to defend their owners. Even if these animals are not of a possessive nature they will also benefit from Chicory together with Red Chestnut (detachment, anguish).

Chicory helps the animal that gets so many cuddles and so much attention from its owners that it ends up thinking it is the 'king' or 'queen' of the castle; and as such has learned to defend its status.

I have also treated animals that needed this remedy not because they had a possessive nature but because they defended their owner from the physical or verbal aggressions of another human. In the majority of these cases the aggressiveness of the animal cannot be solved until its owner's problems have been treated.

Chicory is a component of formulas that address separation anxiety (see Section 5.2, p.111); pseudopregnancy (see Case 6.11, p.186); early maternal rejection of young (see Case 6.3.1, p.154); the arrival of a baby (see Section 5.3, p.113); maternal aggressiveness (see Section 5.1.2, p.107); territorial, possessive and redirected aggressiveness (see Section 5.1.3, p.108); and defecation and urination in inappropriate places (see Section 5.6, p.118).

This remedy also deals with retained accumulations, whether they be liquids (water, urine, blood), fat or faeces.

Local application

As a cream or Aloe Vera gel, Chicory is used in mastitis, mammary tumours and skin accumulations of different natures (see Case 7.9, p.208).

Application to humans

Key words: Selfishly possessive.

Chicory people have trouble loving without imposing conditions and without expecting anything in return. They often claim that they give more love than they receive. Concern for their loved ones is self-centred. This love is sometimes critical, manipulative, dominant, controlling, obstinate, intrusive, selective and involves blackmailing or creating guilt; all these are mechanisms that are sometimes unconscious and which are intended to emotionally wipe out the other person. Underlying these emotional strategies is a deep emotional insufficiency combined with an excessively possessive character that prompts fear of being abandoned or left out and fear of emotional loneliness.

Normally, Chicory people feel self-pity and are easily offended when they do not get what they want by means of their emotional strategies. They frequently respond to this with anger and resentment.

Their self-centredness and demands for attention are sometimes excessive and constant. If this is so, the action of Chicory (possessiveness) should be reinforced with Heather (seeking attention).

4.9 Clematis (Clematis vitalba)

Those who are dreamy, drowsy, not fully awake, no great interest in life. Quiet people, not really happy in their present circumstances, living more in the future than in the present; living in hopes of happier times, when their ideals may come true. In illness some make little or no effort to get well, and in certain cases may even look forward to death, in hope of better times; or maybe, meeting again some beloved one whom they have lost. (Bach 1936)

Application to animals

Key words: Disconnection (TP). Lack of attention (E.B.). Lethargy (TP).

Oral application

Clematis (disconnection) is one of the five components of the Rescue Remedy and its purpose is to help overcome feelings of weakness and emotional paralysis.

It is useful in preventing or treating loss of consciousness due to illness (stroke, seizure), mistreatment, being run over by a car, a fall or a contusion (see Case 6.10.7, p.181).

Clematis is one of the remedies necessary for treating an animal during learning periods, whether it is learning new behavioural guidelines or trying to change habits that entail behavioural problems. It is also useful for the animal that displays a state of lethargy, sometimes as a result of chronic stress.

Local application

As a cream or Aloe Vera gel Clematis is used for all tissues that have necrosis due to insufficient blood circulation. Some animals have this problem in the peripheral tissues of the ears when suffering from Leishmaniasis (see Case 7.6, p.202).

Clematis is useful in the treatment of burns and scarred areas. After a surgical incision the tissues around the wound lose a lot of sensitivity and are energetically weakened.

In general, Clematis is suitable for any area of the body that presents loss of sensitivity.

Application to humans

KEY WORDS: Dreamer. Absent-minded.

Clematis people lack interest in the real world and are therefore lonely and quiet, living in a world of their own. They are also introverted, sensitive and creative (some artists use their Clematis side to their advantage by expressing it through creativity).

Their lack of interest in outside affairs makes Clematis people dreamy, distracted and forgetful. Fantasy constantly wanders through their minds, easily distracting them from their daily tasks and duties. As a result, they often have difficulty in concentrating and have poor memory. Their memory is selective; it records only what interests them. They may have learning problems as a result.

Their lack of connection to the real world and lack of being 'here and now' consumes a lot of energy, hence their fatigue and need for a lot of sleep. Clematis is also used frequently as a remedy for energy input, allowing the person to connect with the present moment. Clematis people normally live in the future, longing for better times but making no effort to achieve them.

This remedy is widely used in teenagers. Teenagers tend to escape from reality, sinking into fantasy worlds that they create from cinema or television. Thus, they delay their emotional maturity, unwilling to assume the obligations of everyday life.

4.10 Crab Apple (Malus pumila)

This is the remedy of cleansing.

For those who feel as if they had something not quite clean about themselves.

Often it is something of apparently little importance: in others there may be more serious disease which is almost disregarded compared to the one thing on which they concentrate.

In both types they are anxious to be free from the one particular thing which is greatest in their minds and which seems so essential to them that it should be cured.

They become despondent if treatment fails.

Being a cleanser, this remedy purifies wounds if the patient has reason to believe that some poison has entered which must be drawn out. (Bach 1936)

Application to animals

KEY WORDS: Impurity (TP). Cleanse (E.B.). Obstruction (TP).

ORAL APPLICATION

Crab Apple is essential in any elimination (diarrhoea, vomiting), cleansing (of poisoning, rotten food), obstruction (constipation) or purification process carried out by the animal's physical body. It is also used for any infectious condition (cold, kennel cough, Leishmaniasis, etc.). While it should never replace veterinary treatment, it can complement it.

If, while taking an oral treatment, any cutaneous or self-cleansing symptoms appear, it is recommended that Crab Apple (impurity) be added to the formula.

Local application

In the form of a cream or Aloe Vera gel Crab Apple (cleanse) is used for abscesses, lumps, infections (of the skin, anal glands, etc.), wounds, sores, mastitis, nodules, stings, burns, cysts, traumatisms, warts and skin diseases in general (see Case 7.2, p.195, Case 7.3, p.196 and Case 7.9, p.208). Crab Apple is essential for treating skin allergies (see Case 7.1, p.193).

In the form of eye-drops it is used to treat infectious and/or allergic conjunctivitis and inflammation of the third eyelid (see Chapter 9).

For otitis, use a sterile saline solution as the formula's diluent vehicle (see Chapter 9, p.235).

Application to humans

KEY WORDS: Feeling of mental or physical impurity.

Physical imperfections generate rejection, disgust or embarrassment in a Crab Apple person. They are methodical, meticulous and obsessive, especially with respect to issues of orderliness and cleanliness. Crab Apple is indispensable for those that are obsessed with having a slim body (anorexia, bulimia) or obsessed with small physical details (a pimple, a slightly crooked nose, etc.). People in this state believe that everybody will notice the physical detail that they think makes them look ugly.

Crab Apple people are also fastidious; they do not like to shake hands, drink from glasses in bars or be around people with colds.

Some people have arrived at a Crab Apple state because they have suffered a major trauma such as rape or abuse in their life. This generates a feeling of being 'dirty'. In these cases you should also include Star of Bethlehem (trauma) in the formula.

Rescue Cream was commercialized after Dr Bach's death; the Rescue Cream contains the five flowers of Rescue Remedy plus Crab Apple. The manufacturers recommend applying it when there is a superficial trauma, such as burns, stings, sores, psoriasis, infections, and so on. Although this cream has proven effective in the emergency situations mentioned above, other more specific formulas can be found throughout this book.

4.11 Elm (Ulmus procera)

Those who are doing good work, are following the calling of their life and who hope to do something of importance, and this often for the benefit of humanity.

At times there may be periods of depression when they feel that the task they have undertaken is too difficult, and not within the power of a human being. (Bach 1936)

Application to animals

KEY WORDS: Being overwhelmed (TP). Pain (R.O.).

ORAL APPLICATION

Elm is sometimes associated with animals' stress by Bach Flower Therapists, because in humans it is characteristic of overwhelmed, stressed-out people, exhausted and depressed when they feel they cannot cope with self-imposed events or activities. Because any emergency situation may involve a certain degree of being overwhelmed, animals can also benefit from Elm (overwhelmed). However, in the canine world stress mainly arises when the animal is subject to a state of constant alert and should therefore be treated with Rock Rose (panic) and Star of Bethlehem (trauma).

Elm is useful in cases of secondary aggressiveness (see Section 5.1.4, p.109) where the animal has an aggressive reaction which may continue after the injury and pain have disappeared.

Local application

As a cream or Aloe Vera gel, Elm is used to treat abscesses, lumps, contusions and, in general, traumatisms that manifest as pain that is sensitive to touch.

To treat otitis use sterile saline solution as the diluent vehicle (see Chapter 9, p.235).

Application to humans

Key words: Suddenly overwhelmed by responsibilities.

The Elm state is usually temporary and develops when usually competent, responsible and expeditious people are exhausted and feel they cannot continue to deal with the issues and concerns that come up in their lives. This comes as a result of accepting too much work for a long period of time without taking into consideration their own personal needs. They become depressed and exhausted, with a temporary loss of self-esteem.

Due to their high expectations of themselves and their perfectionism, people in an Elm state are mentally inflexible. Their belief that they are essential to their company or society puts a lot of pressure on them, which is usually the trigger for their stress. They find delegation very difficult, and if we add to this the fact that they often have an idealized image of themselves, it is easy to see that they will eventually be overwhelmed by the responsibilities they have taken on. This will trigger a high level of stress and temporary doubt in their abilities, as well as anxiety, despondency, fatigue and, in some cases, depression.

4.12 Gentian (Gentianella amarella)

Those who are easily discouraged. They may be progressing well in illness or in the affairs of their daily life, but any small delay or hindrance to progress causes doubt and soon disheartens them. (Bach 1936)

Application to animals

Key words: Discouragement (E.B.).

Oral application

Gentian (discouragement) is very useful for those animals that refuse to eat or drink despite the vet not finding any physiological cause that justifies this behaviour. Any animal may manifest this condition, but the majority of cases I have treated have been cats as they are animals of a very sensitive nature. Although Gorse (submission) is the most important remedy for this problem, more satisfactory results are achieved if both the remedies are combined. In other cases it has been necessary to add Wild Rose (apathy) and Clematis (disconnection) for the animal to overcome its state of lethargy.

Remember to take into consideration the states underlying this behaviour, such as fear, panic, trauma or sadness, especially in mistreated and/or abandoned animals.

Local application

No known application.

Application to humans

Key words: Discouragement and pessimism.

Gentian people quickly become discouraged when their ambitions are not fulfilled. They make a mountain out of a molehill because they have a low tolerance for frustration.

It is a good remedy for convalescent people who have been left feeling dejected by a long or recurrent disease. Gentian manages pessimism. People in need of Gentian experience obstacles as failures in all the areas of their life, including family, work and emotional relationships, or in their convalescence. It is their negative expectations that frustrate their success (our mind builds our future reality), and they often surrender ahead of time in any situation. Their motto is 'Why try, if it is going to go wrong anyway?' They tend to find grievances in the situations that affect them. If they are invited to go to the countryside they may reject the invitation as they are convinced it will rain. If they travel, on their return they will say that it was not that great and not worth the money.

Gentian is appropriate for sceptics and those with a very Cartesian mindset who think they can handle everything through reason. They are rational, analytical and often deny their pessimistic behaviour, claiming they are realistic.

4.13 Gorse (Ulex europaeus)

Very great hopelessness, they have given up belief that more can be done for them.

Under persuasion or to please others they may try different treatments, at the same time assuring those around that there is so little hope of relief. (Bach 1936)

Application to animals

KEY WORDS: Submission (TP). Boost to the immune system (P.N.). Resignation (E.B.).

ORAL APPLICATION

Gorse (submission) is the main remedy when treating an animal that refuses to eat or drink despite the absence of a physiological cause that justifies this behaviour. We also use it in some animal shelters (especially those in rural areas where a lot of animals have been used for hunting) when an exhausted animal which has been mistreated, poisoned or run over arrives, and generally in any situation where the animal is very devitalized.

In very debilitated animals, also add Olive (exhaustion) and Centaury (weakness) to the Bach Flower formula. This is relevant for dogs that have been attacked or poisoned (sometimes by hunters if the animal 'was no longer good for hunting'). Also add Mustard (sadness) and Wild Rose (apathy) if these animals retreat into a corner without interacting with their environment.

For its boost to the immune system, Gorse is one of the components of the Leishmaniasis formula (see p.166). It is also part of the formula that treats and prevents colds. In places with cold weather, especially animal shelters located in the mountains where winter temperatures are extreme, it is recommended that cats (the animals most susceptible to catching colds) be treated with the formula that prevents this very contagious condition (see Chapter 9, p.231). In general, Gorse helps in any process that manifests as infection, such as kennel cough (see p.225).

LOCAL APPLICATION

No known application.

Application to humans

KEY WORDS: Loss of hope.

Gorse helps people who have given up fighting because they have lost hope of finding a solution to their problem. This may be due to a chronic disease or simply because they have lost confidence in their own healing resources after trying everything. People in a Gorse (submission) state believe they are doomed to pain and suffering. Their despair is based on the fact that they have tried a thousand things without success. They have suffered so many failures and disappointments that they refuse to continue. This chronic resignation results in blockages that prevent any type of improvement. If there is some improvement they may well discontinue the treatment, arguing that the results are not worth the effort. Some people in a Gorse state expect their situation to be resolved by some form of external help instead of admitting and accepting that healing always comes from within oneself.

4.14 Heather (Calluna vulgaris)

Those who are always seeking the companionship of anyone who may be available, as they find it necessary to discuss their own affairs with others, no matter whom it may be. They are very unhappy if they have to be alone for any length of time. (Bach 1936)

Application to animals

KEY WORDS: Demanding attention (E.B.).

ORAL APPLICATION

Heather is the remedy that helps animals that demand attention constantly. This behaviour should not necessarily be treated; however, there are animals that manifest signs of aggressiveness if they cannot be their owners' centre of attention. This is the case for animals that change their behaviour when a baby arrives home, for the female who rejects her own young (see Case 6.3.1, p.154) and for the animal that has to share space and affection with another animal that has recently arrived at the house. In all of these cases, Heather's (demanding attention) action should be enhanced by Chicory (possessiveness), Beech (intolerance) and Holly (jealousy).

Heather is included in formulas that address separation anxiety (see Section 5.2, p.111), coprophagia (see Section 5.4, p.115), stereotypic behaviour (see Section 5.7, p.120), pseudopregnancy (see Section 5.12, p.130) and the anxiety of the animal that eats everything it finds on the street (see Case 6.5, p.160).

LOCAL APPLICATION

No known application.

Application to humans

KEY WORDS: Self-centred and worried about oneself.

Heather people need to talk about themselves nonstop and do so compulsively. They always choose someone, either known to them or a stranger, to whom to explain their problems or illnesses, exaggerating or lying if necessary about what happens in their life in order to attract more attention or sympathy from the other person. Heather people need others around them because they need to be listened to and not to feel alone. With this attitude they absorb others' energy, continuing to talk to them even if they do not show the slightest interest in listening any further. Heather people find that the best way of communicating is by monologue as they have no interest at all in other people's problems. It is therefore not surprising that those around Heather people flee from their company. This prevents Heather people from receiving the affection and love they long for. Heather is the remedy to enable empathy, the ability to understand and appreciate others' needs.

Underlying this way of being is a severe and profound problem of lack of affection and fear of loneliness that often leads Heather people to be indiscriminate with their relationships, associating themselves emotionally or sexually with anyone. Heather people have demanded attention since they were babies, regardless of whether they received it constantly or not. Their childhood circumstances have not enabled them to satisfy their emotional needs, for example in the case of abandoned children, a cold and harsh family environment, a very large family, and so on.

Their exaggerated self-observation and self-centredness will cause them serious problems with hypochondria.

4.15 Holly (Ilex aquifolium)

For those who are sometimes attacked by thoughts of such kind as jealousy, envy, revenge, suspicion.
For the different forms of vexation.
Within themselves they may suffer much, often when there is no real cause for their unhappiness. (Bach 1936)

Application to animals

KEY WORDS: Jealousy (E.B.). Eruption (TP). Mistrust. Hypersensitivity (E.B.). Rage (E.B.).

ORAL APPLICATION

Holly (jealousy, mistrust) is one of the remedies used in the formulas that treat aggressiveness (see Section 5.1, p.105). Its use should be considered in particular for an animal's preventive treatment before the arrival of a newborn baby to the house. In this case it is recommended that the animal be treated during and after the owner's pregnancy, as in many countries large numbers of dogs and cats have been abandoned or put down for behaving aggressively towards the owner or baby.

Holly is also used in cases where the female rejects her own young due to jealousy (see Case 6.3.1, p.154) and for animals that have to share their home and family with another animal that has just arrived.

Holly is also used in psychological pregnancy (see Section 5.12, p.130). First, it helps in managing the high degree of hypersensitivity that the female dog experiences during this period, and second, it ensures that you avoid aggressiveness if you try to take away any object adopted by the animal as a replacement baby. It is also used to regulate hypersensitivity when the female is in heat (see Chapter 9, p.233) and defecation and urination in inappropriate places (see Section 5.6, p.118), and is one of the components of the kennel cough formula (see p.227).

LOCAL APPLICATION

As a cream or Aloe Vera gel, Holly is used in acute inflammations showing redness and/or itchiness, for example abscesses, skin rashes (eruptions) of an allergic or infectious nature, herpes and mastitis (see Case 7.8, p.206).

Application to humans

> **KEY WORDS**: Envy, jealousy, anger, suspiciousness or desire of revenge.

People in a Holly state are instinctive, very insecure and vulnerable, and are always on the defensive. It is therefore part of the hypersensitivity group. They are offended, irritated and get angry easily and they often blame others for their bad temper. They are also jealous, envious, ill-tempered, spiteful (they have a hard time forgiving others) and suspicious. In many cases their suspiciousness and jealousy have no real basis in reality, and this will cause them serious difficulties in their relationships. Ultimately they favour stormy relationships and emotional break-ups that deepen their anger and rage, unleashing their desire for revenge, which results in physical or verbal aggressiveness.

Behind Holly behaviours there are always people with a deep emotional need who experience all aspects of their life with a lot of insecurity and low self-esteem. In short, they are people who lose their capacity to love in order to make way for outbursts of rage and anger directed towards others.

Holly emotions in all their different aspects (hate, anger, envy, jealousy, revenge, suspiciousness, etc.) are very present in modern life. This remedy integrates these feelings and emotions into our lives positively instead of repressing them or covering them up.

Ancient medicines such as Traditional Chinese Medicine have shown that the emotion of hatred is directly related to diseases of the digestive tract, especially the liver meridian.

4.16 Honeysuckle (Lonicera caprifolium)

Those who live much in the past, perhaps a time of great happiness, or memories of a lost friend, or ambitions which have not come true. They do not expect further happiness such as they have had. (Bach 1936)

Application to animals

KEY WORDS: Melancholy (E.B.). Regression (TP).

ORAL APPLICATION

Honeysuckle (regression) and Clematis (disconnection) are used in animals with infantilism – a behaviour or body language that does not correspond to their current age. A clear example of infantilism is the adult dog that still adopts the 'frog' position when stretched out on the floor or manifests other aspects of behaviour typical of a puppy or a younger animal.

Honeysuckle (melancholy) helps the dog that is sad because its owner has died. Some dogs spend a long time lying by the front door of the house waiting for their owner to return. There have been cases in rural areas where dogs have remained prostrate for hours in front of the cemetery or place the owner has been buried without showing any interest in moving from the spot. The remedy is also helpful for the animal that expresses sadness at the absence of another animal that used to live with it.

LOCAL APPLICATION

No known application.

Application to humans

KEY WORDS: Homesickness. Living in the past.

Essentially, the Honeysuckle remedy treats our unresolved emotional issues with our past, whether pleasant or unpleasant, recent or distant. The Honeysuckle state may be reached because the present does not interest us or because of past traumatic events that linger in our minds and prevent us from living in the present. People in a Honeysuckle state live immersed in nostalgia. They do not expect to find happiness like they experienced in the past again.

This remedy is very useful for people who, for various reasons, have been separated from their families and are living with grief, for example those who are moving town or country for studies or work, couples who have recently separated, or those who have lost a loved one. In short, they are people who need to work on their emotional detachment. It is also highly recommended for elderly people who remember their past with nostalgia, convinced that the future holds nothing better for them.

Honeysuckle is very important for people who have not changed the way they dress, their hairstyle or their make-up for many years. It is also for children who still have a pacifier in their mouth, despite this behaviour not corresponding to their age, or for those who still suck their thumb, yearning for the pacifier.

Honeysuckle should be considered in any situation likely to be experienced with nostalgia and melancholy, for example retirement, abandonment, orphanhood, migration, and so on.

4.17 Hornbeam (Carpinus betulus)

For those who feel that they have not sufficient strength, mentally or physically, to carry the burden of life placed upon them; the affairs of every day seem too much for them to accomplish, though they generally succeed in fulfilling their task.

For those who believe that some part, of mind or body, needs to be strengthened before they can easily fulfil their work. (Bach 1936)

Application to animals

KEY WORDS: Weakness (TP). Energy. Laxity (TP).

ORAL APPLICATION

No known application.

LOCAL APPLICATION

As a cream or Aloe Vera gel, Hornbeam (weakness) helps animals that have suffered an injury or a stroke with paralysis of a limb by providing energy to the weakened area (see Chapter 9).

As eye-drops it provides energy where there are peripheral corneal ulcers.

Application to humans

KEY WORDS: Fatigue. Mental fatigue. Discouraged.

Hornbeam people find it difficult to cope with everyday tasks or problems. They normally experience them as redundant and boring. Their mental laziness hinders them in 'starting-up' but when they finally do so they manage to perform the proposed task.

They experience routine and monotony in a very negative manner. The Hornbeam state often disappears when they substitute the everyday activity that they experience as an obligation with another that brings distraction or fun. Hornbeam therefore helps manage boredom.

Hornbeam fatigue is a tiredness that arises mentally. For this reason, the remedy helps fight the feeling that everyone has experienced: the lack of mental energy to face a new day, especially if it is Monday morning. Fatigue starts when we get up and think of all the everyday situations that await us and which we would like to postpone. Everything that was once a pleasure has become an obligation. People in a Hornbeam state doubt if they will be able yet again to endure another boring day without incentives. Therefore they start slowly, delaying any obligation as much as possible. In the Hornbeam state there is no feeling of exhaustion due to suffering as in the case of Olive. The person has a mental fatigue that is rapidly somatized in the form of physical fatigue. It is a type of tiredness that disappears just as quickly when a more interesting or different activity or plan arises.

4.18 Impatiens (Impatiens glandulifera)

Those who are quick in thought and action and who wish all things to be done without hesitation or delay. When ill they are anxious for a hasty recovery.

They find it very difficult to be patient with people who are slow, as they consider it wrong and a waste of time, and they will endeavour to make such people quicker in all ways.

They often prefer to work and think alone, so that they can do everything at their own speed. (Bach 1936)

Application to animals

KEY WORDS: Acceleration (TP).

ORAL APPLICATION

Impatiens (acceleration) helps the restless, nervous and hyperactive animal that moves from one place to another without stopping and is never comfortable anywhere. It is also for the stressed animal that lives in a very small space, such as an animal shelter, cage, and so on.

This remedy is part of the formula used to treat separation anxiety (see Section 5.2, p.111), coprophagia (see Section 5.4, p.115), stereotypic behaviour (see Section 5.7, p.120) and the anxiety of the animal that eats everything it finds on the street.

Local application

As a cream or Aloe Vera gel, consider using Impatiens in skin irritations or allergies that manifest as pruritus. Also consider it in otitis and other pains that involve swelling.

Application to humans

Key words: Impatience.

Impatiens people are competent and effective. They are easily irritated and frustrated when working with slow-paced people and therefore prefer to work alone. They want everything done at once. They are energetic, but their impulsiveness, impatience and nervous tension sweep them in to living at an accelerated pace. They act, think and speak quickly, regardless of whether they have few or many tasks to complete. They are always in the fast lane, even if they are not in a hurry, and this makes it difficult for them to go into depth in the situations they encounter in life. In short, it makes it difficult for them to learn and mature.

As a result of their impatience and acceleration, Impatiens people have difficulties in waiting for someone to finish talking or carrying out a task. They find it difficult to wait their turn and end up talking over the other person's voice or abruptly finishing a sentence that the other person 'had in hand'. Impatiens people have no time for anyone, including themselves.

Their great irritability easily provokes rage attacks that disappear just as quickly. They usually arrive at their appointments either too early (due to their impatience) or late (to avoid having to wait or because they were busy doing other things). Time 'flies' for them.

They are not really in a hurry; the fact is that they do not know how to do things at a slow pace. If they do not show their inner impatience through their words they do so through their gestures: drumming with their fingers, constant leg movements, rocking in a chair, and so on.

Impatiens is one of the five components of Rescue Remedy and its purpose is to bring calmness and relieve restlessness and anxiety in specific moments of emergency.

4.19 Larch (Larix deciduas)

For those who do not consider themselves as good or capable as those around them, who expect failure, who feel that they will never be a success, and so do not venture or make a strong enough attempt to succeed. (Bach 1936)

Application to animals

KEY WORDS: Disability (TP).

ORAL APPLICATION

Larch (disability) increases the confidence and self-esteem of the animal during any learning process. Remember also to consider Cerato (dispersion), Clematis (facilitates attention) and Chestnut Bud (learning process) in these processes. The synergistic interaction between these four remedies allows the animal to process the new behavioural guidelines faster and assimilate the information from the rest of the Flower Remedies in the formula more easily. It is therefore a common remedy in formulas when training and/or educating an animal, or when trying to change inappropriate habits or patterns that may lead to behavioural problems. These four remedies are helpful for the canine trainer, behaviourist or Bach Flower Therapist in their work with animals.

LOCAL APPLICATION

As a cream or Aloe Vera gel, Larch is part of the formula that rehabilitates the area of the body that is unable to function or move correctly after a traumatism.

Application to humans

Key words: Lack of confidence. Disability.

People in a Larch state invent thousands of excuses in order to avoid tasks they believe they are unable to carry out. They hinder their own progress using various elaborate and rational arguments to justify themselves. Larch people feel inferior to others and therefore do not take action or any risks. At the same time they expect to fail because this will serve as an excuse to justify their 'not taking action'. Some Larch people feel that they are capable of doing things well but refuse to admit so in order to avoid the risk of failure. In others, not wishing to mature or take on responsibilities underlies their 'not taking action'.

Larch is very useful for anyone who shows a lack of confidence before any specific important event, such as exams, interviews, driving tests, and so on.

There are personal situations that lead to a Larch state, especially during those life stages when the person is growing or maturing. At those times individuals must acquire self-confidence and a solid assessment of their skills and attitudes, that is, a good level of self-esteem. Consider the following examples:

- Children with overprotective parents or teachers who are excessively critical or rigid. This strictness imprints on the children the belief that 'I am not capable.' It prevents children from taking the initiative by imposing a sense of fear of failure or getting hurt. The parents claim the children are too young or criticize how they carry things out.

- Children who have a gifted brother or other close family member and are constantly being compared to him or her by relatives, teachers or themselves.

- Children who have not been treated and educated through positive reinforcement, that is, with praise and enhancement of their positive qualities.

4.20 Mimulus (Mimulus guttatus)

Fear of worldly things, illness, pain, accidents, poverty, of dark, of being alone, of misfortune. The fears of everyday life. These people quietly and secretly bear their dread, they do not freely speak of it to others. (Bach 1936)

Application to animals

KEY WORDS: Fear (E.B.).

ORAL APPLICATION

Mimulus (fear) is one of the remedies used to help the animal that is fearful by nature. Animals may associate a dangerous situation they have experienced with a related object. For example, an animal whose previous owner mistreated it with a broom may get scared each time its new owner starts sweeping. The animal's brain, specifically its limbic system, has made a direct association between broom and danger. We recommend Mimulus for this kind of fear in animals, and we always suggest considering Rock Rose (panic) too because the fear may be more terror than phobia in some cases.

LOCAL APPLICATION

No known application.

Application to humans

KEY WORDS: Fear of familiar things.

Mimulus people are usually shy and reserved, uncommunicative in public and blush easily. They are usually very sensitive to being rejected. Anxious by nature, they avoid crowds of people and very noisy places.

Phobias are generally covered by Mimulus, but if they experience a real situation associated with their phobia, they should also be treated with Rock Rose (panic). These two remedies are an excellent combination to enable the Mimulus personality to confront with courage and strength those situations which they experience with fear and terror, for example stage fright, having to speak before an audience, fear of surgery, fear of the dentist, fear of flying, and so on.

Mimulus is associated with an evasive personality and corresponds to people who may have the following characteristics: sensitive, introverted, shy, bashful, vulnerable, very insecure, reserved, repressed, fearful, apprehensive, anxious, nervous, hypochondriac, obsessive and easily offended.

4.21 Mustard (Sinapis arvensis)

Those who are liable to times of gloom, or even despair, as though a cold dark cloud overshadowed them and hid the light and the joy of life. It may not be possible to give any reason or explanation for such attacks.

Under these conditions it is almost impossible to appear happy or cheerful. (Bach 1936)

Application to animals

Key words: Depression (TP). Sadness (E.B.).

Oral application

Mustard (sadness) helps the dog that is sad because its owner has died. Some spend a long time lying behind the front door of the house waiting for their owner to return. In rural areas there have been cases where dogs have spent hours lying by the entrance of the cemetery or place where their owner has been buried, without any interest in moving from the spot. It should also be administered to animals expressing sadness due to the absence of another animal with which they lived.

LOCAL APPLICATION

No known application.

Application to humans

KEY WORDS: Sadness. Melancholy.

People in need of Mustard live submerged in deep sadness. This negative mood cannot always be justified by one specific reason and is not the prelude to a depressive syndrome in all cases. However, if the Mustard state lasts too long people can fall into a deep depression where they may also feel melancholy, lack of pleasure, suffering, lack of motivation and concentration, apathy, isolation and lack of libido. This is the result of an interior emptiness that prevents them from enjoying any situation in their life.

4.22 Oak (Quercus robur)

For those who are struggling and fighting strongly to get well, or in connection with the affairs of their daily life. They will go on trying one thing after another, though their case may seem hopeless.

They will fight on. They are discontented with themselves if illness interferes with their duties or helping others.

They are brave people, fighting against great difficulties, without loss of hope or effort. (Bach 1936)

Application to animals

KEY WORDS: Obsession.

Oral application

At present, the administration of this remedy in animals is under study.

Oak follows a pattern of obsession and is being tested together with Rock Water (resistance to change) in persistent behavioural problems.

Local application

No known application.

Application to humans

Key words: Fighting spirit. Tenacity.

Oak people, like the tree, are of a strong, vigorous, resistant, generous and noble nature, and shelter all the 'creatures of the forest'.

Oak people are the backbone of the family. They try their best, fight endlessly to help others and are motivated by a sense of duty and obligation. They never complain and, although they may live through very difficult situations, they will not stop fighting. When they fall ill, they do not allow themselves to stop or rest. They do not pay attention to what their bodies tell them and they soldier on, impatient to improve as soon as possible. They are able neither to ask for help nor to accept it. For them it would be a sign of weakness and vulnerability that would make them dependent. They are workaholic (they feel obliged), demanding a lot from themselves and pushing their limits, even at times when they have no more strength, until they finally suffer from a heart attack, stroke, nervous breakdown, great dejection or depression.

Behind this lifestyle based on struggle and persistent work, some Oak people hide their fear of poverty and therefore some of them are austere.

As far as showing affection is concerned, Oak people may have communication problems with their partners, children and relatives because they mistake sensitivity for sentimentality. They are often disconnected from the emotional world and from their own limitations. Their way of expressing love to their loved ones is to make sure they are not lacking anything.

This state is also typical in people who have lived through a post-war period suffering hunger and as a result have become determined fighters.

4.23 Olive (Olea europaea)

Those who have suffered much mentally or physically and are so exhausted and weary that they feel they have no more strength to make any effort. Daily life is hard work for them, without pleasure. (Bach 1936)

Application to animals

KEY WORDS: Exhaustion (TP). Revitalizing.

ORAL APPLICATION

Olive (exhaustion) is a remedy which provides energy for the exhausted animal after experiencing a situation of suffering, such as malnutrition due to abandonment, devitalization by illness, being run over, attempted poisoning, mistreatment, visits to the vet, preoperative and postoperative procedures, and so on (see Chapter 9). It is a remedy that also helps an animal that is dying.

If the animal is mistreated for a long period of time, its stress level moves from acute to chronic. When the physiological substances involved in the response to the situation in question act continuously, the excess of cortisol causes side effects in the animal. Olive will bring energy to the adrenal glands, which are in charge of secreting cortisol into the bloodstream (see Section 5.8, p.121).

Olive is one of the components of the formula that helps dogs with Leishmaniasis or chronic stress.

According to the work carried out in Traditional Chinese Medicine and Bach Flowers by Pablo Noriega (2006), using Olive together with Gorse helps enhance the correct functioning of the immune system (see 'Colds', p.231).

Local application

As a cream or Aloe Vera gel, Olive, together with Hornbeam (local energy), provides energy directly to severely debilitated areas.

Application to humans

Key words: Exhaustion. Lack of energy. Lack of vitality.

An Olive state is reached after a long period of stress, study, overwork, personal difficulties, significant lack of sleep, major infection, surgery, childbirth, chronic illness or long-term care of a sick person, or simply after a situation where there has been a lot of physical, emotional or psychological suffering. People who have experienced any of these situations enter a state of extreme exhaustion after using all of their body's energy reserves.

Olive's severe exhaustion is not solved by extra sleep because it is a weariness that comes from a situation of suffering or having worn oneself out. This remedy manages both physical and mental exhaustion.

Taking Olive quickly redirects available energy. However, if we insist on working beyond our means, there will not be enough energy available and then Olive will act 'wisely' and connect us with our need to rest and limit ourselves.

According to the work of Pablo Noriega (2006), Olive is a great invigorator of the kidney meridian. When this meridian is irregular (as a result of fear or panic episodes in the person) great exhaustion occurs. Consider this remedy when a person needs dialysis.

4.24 Pine (Pinus sylvestris)

For those who blame themselves. Even when successful they think they could have done better, and are never content with their efforts or the results. They are hard working and suffer much from the faults they attach to themselves.

Sometimes if there is any mistake it is due to another, but they will claim responsibility even for that. (Bach 1936)

Application to animals

KEY WORDS: None.

ORAL APPLICATION
No known application.

LOCAL APPLICATION
No known application.

Application to humans

KEY WORDS: Self-accusation. Feelings of guilt.

People in a Pine state feel they are unworthy and lack merit. They act in a humble manner and are always asking for forgiveness and permission for everything.

They are very perfectionist and self-demanding, and cannot tolerate making mistakes. They tend towards undermining themselves. Even when they are successful they think they could have done better. They are never satisfied with their efforts nor with the results they obtain and sometimes blame themselves for mistakes that they did not make.

Many of them maintain difficult and at times violent relationships which involve a lot of suffering; this is usually an unconscious means of self-punishment for feeling 'unworthy', and for 'not deserving a better life' as they believe they are to blame for everything. Generally, the origin of this model they have chosen can be found in an incapacitating childhood with very puritanical, critical, rigid, excessively dominant, cold or tyrannical parents. In short, as children these people were educated with strictness, punishment and disapproval, and they in turn accepted the responsibility and blame for everything that happened around them.

There are Pine states that are temporary – for example, the feeling of forgetting to congratulate someone on his or her birthday, making an unwise/tactless/indiscreet/unfortunate comment to someone, or breaking a glass when dining with friends.

4.25 Red Chestnut (Aesculus carnea)

For those who find it difficult not to be anxious for other people.
Often they have ceased to worry about themselves, but for those of whom they are fond they may suffer much, frequently anticipating that some unfortunate thing may happen to them. (Bach 1936)

Application to animals

KEY WORDS: Detachment.

ORAL APPLICATION

In canines, Red Chestnut (detachment) helps the female manage the level of anguish experienced during pseudopregnancy (see Section 5.12, p.130). Red Chestnut is also recommended for puppies that are being weaned (between one and two months of age).

LOCAL APPLICATION

No known application.

Application to humans

KEY WORDS: Anguish felt for others.

Red Chestnut deals with the anticipatory and disproportionate fear of something happening to a loved one. Many mothers experience the Red Chestnut emotion when their children leave on a journey. They ask them to call as soon as they reach their destination; only then will they relax. The same happens when they go out at night; the mother cannot sleep until her children return home, fearing that something might happen to them.

People in this state worry too much about others, especially about family and closest friends. Normally this causes Red Chestnut people and those around them to live in constant anxiety.

It is important to point out that beneath Red Chestnut people's phobic fear, projected onto their loved ones, lies their own difficulty when experiencing fear firsthand. They therefore feel the need to shift responsibility for that fear onto others: 'They are the reason of my fear, not me' or 'I need you around me to feel better.'

Red Chestnut people are excessively concerned about others and very little about themselves. This attitude leads them to unconsciously avoid addressing their own problems because they are afraid to connect with themselves.

There are Red Chestnut states induced by a previous traumatic experience. Some people also experience the Red Chestnut emotion towards belongings or animals. Sometimes the anxiety inherent to this state can be transmitted from the owner to the animal, hence the need to treat the animals at the same time as the owners with this remedy.

4.26 Rock Rose (Helianthemum nummularium)

The rescue remedy. The remedy of emergency for cases where there even appears no hope. In accident or sudden illness, or when the patient is very frightened or terrified, or if the condition is serious enough to cause great fear to those around. If the patient is not conscious the lips may be moistened with the remedy. Other remedies in addition may also be required, as, for example, if there is unconsciousness, which is a deep, sleepy state, Clematis; if there is torture, Agrimony, and so on. (Bach 1936)

Application to animals

Key words: Panic (E.B.). Paralysis (TP). Terror (E.B.).

Oral application

Rock Rose (panic) will form part of any formula that helps animals which have been mistreated, abandoned, run over or stressed out, and for those that have experienced a traumatic event with after effects of panic or terror. This post-traumatic syndrome can leave an imprint on the animal that makes it difficult to adjust to a new situation, such as arriving at an animal shelter, a new home, and so on. It also helps animals that hyperventilate in the face of a specific stressful situation. In this situation the remedy should be administered in direct application at high frequency until the hyperventilation has ceased.

Rock Rose (panic) is the main remedy used to treat animals of a fearful nature and those that have experienced any of the situations mentioned above. Also use in the case of animals that do not want to leave the house after the loss of their 'housemate', for example if their housemate has been put down because of an illness or has been 'relocated' to another home (see Case 6.10.9, p.184). Consider using this remedy when animals have to travel separately from their owners by any means of transport that requires them to be inside a cage. It is also useful for treating those animals that become stressed when they go to the vet or when they hear a loud noise (see Chapter 9). Rock Rose is one of the components used to treat fear-induced aggressiveness (see Section 5.1.1, p.106).

Rock Rose panic can also paralyze an animal (see Case 6.10.6, p.180; Case 6.10.7, p.181; Case 6.10.8, p.183; and Case 6.10.9, p.184).

LOCAL APPLICATION

As a cream or Aloe Vera gel and together with other remedies, Rock Rose (sudden paralysis) has been used to treat the paralysis of a part of the animal's body (face or limbs). This remedy has proven effective both for paralysis due to a specific cause, such as a stroke (see Case 6.10.7, p.181), and for paralysis without an apparent cause (see Case 6.10.8, p.183).

Application to humans

KEY WORDS: Terror. Panic.

Dr Bach initially called Rock Rose 'Emergency Remedy'.

This remedy is administered in critical situations of terror and helplessness. It also deals with the residual panic associated with past traumas. Sometimes this panic emerges in the form of nightmares. Rock Rose is one of the most important remedies for anxiety and panic attacks. The panic may physically block or paralyze a person. It is useful for people who have lost the ability to speak after experiencing a very shocking situation where they were seized by terror and panic (e.g. rape, witnessing unpleasant events). In these cases Star of Bethlehem (trauma) together with Rock Rose and Sweet Chestnut (extreme anguish) must also be administered.

There are also individuals with a Rock Rose personality. Rock Rose people live with an unconscious fear of all things physical and are prone to panic in circumstances that for others would not be so alarming. Their hypersensitivity to external stimuli makes it relatively easily for them to be startled and allows any unexpected event or change to be experienced as a borderline risk situation. This threatens their physical integrity by somaticizing as shivers, sweaty palms, diarrhoea, loss of sphincter control, and so on.

4.27 Rock Water

Those who are very strict in their way of living; they deny themselves many of the joys and pleasures of life because they consider it might interfere with their work.

They are hard masters to themselves. They wish to be well and strong and active, and will do anything which they believe will keep them so. They hope to be examples which will appeal to others who may then follow their ideas and be better as a result. (Bach 1936)

Application to animals

KEY WORDS: Hardness (TP). Resistance to change.

ORAL APPLICATION

Currently we recommend using Rock Water (resistance to change) in animals that display a persistent anomalous behaviour such as separation anxiety. The canine trainer and Flower Therapist Antonio Paramio has discovered that there are anomalous behaviours in animals that are not the result of a Walnut (adaptation) problem, but rather a problem of resistance to change due to behavioural patterns that are very well established due to the dog's age and personal history (Paramio 2009). In addition, if, as Antonio Paramio claims, dogs are indeed quite obsessive-compulsive in their behaviours and routines, it is easy to understand why Rock Water should be added to a dog's treatment, regardless of the behavioural problem it has. The aim of the treatment is to achieve a behavioural change and in order to do so it is necessary to eliminate resistance to that change.

LOCAL APPLICATION

As a cream or Aloe Vera gel, and together with other remedies, Rock Water (hardness) has proven effective in treating nodules of unknown aetiology (see Case 7.9, p.208). The success of this remedy in treating physical formations that appear to be hard (lumps, superficial cysts, warts, etc.) is undergoing research.

In eye-drops (sterile saline solution) Rock Water is used to improve ocular dryness as, according to the work of Pablo Noriega (2006), this remedy boosts the formation of liquids.

Application to humans

> **KEY WORDS**: Self-repression. Desire to be taken as a role model. Moral strictness.

Rock Water people have important ideals and firm principles and wish to be seen as a role model. They are anchored to a traditional way of life, to conventionalism and stability. In short, they are resistant to change. They may have high spiritual and philosophical ideals and excessive moral laws that lead them to puritanism, fanaticism, perfectionism, self-discipline and an excessive self-demand and self-repression. These attitudes do not allow them to live a life full of joy, pleasure, spontaneity and magic. On the contrary, their way of living is repressive, strict, rigid, static, boring and very conventional.

The kinds of people we find in this state include: sectarians and religious extremists of a very rigid morality; those who are saints and martyrs by 'vocation'; moralists; those who follow very strict eating habits and lifestyles (extreme followers of vegetarian or macrobiotic diets, anti-smoking, anti-alcohol, anti-sexuality, elite athletes, gym addicts, top models); and people with a very strict monotonous timetable where there is no room for improvisation and where everything has to be planned and timed. In short, they are stiff and rigid people who often give up all that deviates them from their goals.

Underlying this behavioural pattern is their search for recognition and to be seen as a role model.

4.28 Scleranthus (Scleranthus annus)

Those who suffer much from being unable to decide between two things, first one seeming right then the other.

They are usually quiet people, and bear their difficulty alone, as they are not inclined to discuss it with others. (Bach 1936)

Application to animals

KEY WORDS: Cyclicity (TP). Instability (TP).

Oral application

Scleranthus (instability) is used in animals that suffer from travel sickness.

Scleranthus is part of the Leishmaniasis formula because of the cyclicity manifested in this illness.

Also consider using this remedy as a hormone stabilizer for a female that is in heat (see Chapter 9, p.233).

Local application

No known application.

Application to humans

Key words: Indecision. Instability.

Scleranthus is used in people or states dominated by indecision, insecurity and changeability. Despite doubting their decisions, Scleranthus people almost never ask others for advice. They debate with themselves in silence when deciding between two possible options.

The Scleranthus personality is very emotionally unstable and undergoes frequent and rapid emotional changes – love–hate, joy–sadness, calmness–aggressiveness, and so on – manifesting mood swings which in extreme cases may result in bipolarity.

Scleranthus people are highly changeable. They start several things at the same time but do not finish any of them. They are also very contradictory. They may make plans to do something, for example go to the cinema, and then soon after go back on their word. They are seen as informal and changeable people. They are also obsessive and very chaotic in their way of thinking, doing or expressing themselves. This results in anxiety, impaired concentration and memory, and difficulty falling asleep.

4.29 Star of Bethlehem (Ornithogalum umbellatum)

For those in great distress under conditions which for a time produce great unhappiness.

The shock of serious news, the loss of someone dear, the fright following an accident, and such like.

For those who for a time refuse to be consoled, this remedy brings comfort. (Bach 1936)

Application to animals

Key words: Cicatrizant (R.O.) Energetic connector (R.O.). Repair (R.O.). Resistance (TP). Traumatic shock (E.B.).

Oral application

Star of Bethlehem, used together with Rock Rose (panic), is necessary for alleviating the effects of a traumatic shock, such as abandonment, mistreatment, accidents, arrival at a shelter (in animals manifesting fear), firework celebrations, visits to the vet, and preoperative and postoperative periods (see Chapter 9). Consider using this remedy with animals that are very shocked and do not want to leave the house any more after the death of their owner or companion animal, for example if another animal has been put down due to illness or relocated to another home.

Local application

As a cream or Aloe Vera gel, and together with other remedies, Star of Bethlehem is used to help cicatrize a cut, wound, bite, sore, and so on. It is also applied in synergy with other remedies for any type of traumatism: accidents, bone fractures, contusions, hemiplegia, bites, and so on. It can be used to treat inflammation and/or infection of the anal glands and mastitis (see Chapter 9, pp.233–234). Star of Bethlehem repairs (at an energetical level) any disconnections that may occur in the physical body of the animal when it experiences a traumatic situation.

Application to humans

KEY WORDS: For the effects of a shock.

This remedy treats the unresolved aspects of a traumatic experience, be they physical (accidents, contusions, bone fractures, illness, etc.) or psychological (death of a loved one, emotional separation, witnessing an unpleasant event, mistreatment, rape, etc.). It does not matter if the traumatic experience is recent or belongs to the past, or if the person remembers or has forgotten it. If the trauma has not been dealt with, the person will experience energetic blockages that affect his or her current life and may cause physical or psychological problems (visions, recurring memories or thoughts, traumatic dreams, obsessions, phobias, panic, etc.). Phobias and panic should also be treated with Rock Rose (panic).

Star of Bethlehem is one of the five components of Rescue Remedy and its aim is to alleviate the effects of a shock.

4.30 Sweet Chestnut (Castanea saliva)

For those moments which happen to some people when the anguish is so great as to seem to be unbearable.

When the mind or body feels as if it had borne to the uttermost limit of its endurance, and that now it must give way.

When it seems there is nothing but destruction and annihilation left to face. (Bach 1936)

Application to animals

KEY WORDS: Extreme anguish (E.B.).

ORAL APPLICATION

Sweet Chestnut (extreme anguish) is of great help in dealing with the extreme suffering and anguish that often accompany specific and extreme stressful situations, for example in the cases of animals that are run over, abandoned, mistreated, undergoing surgery or attacked by another animal. It is recommended that you consider this remedy when an animal is very distressed after the death of its owner or an animal that lived with it.

Sweet Chestnut is also used for animals that hyperventilate when they hear loud noises (e.g. firework celebrations), when going to the vet, or when they have to travel separately from their owners in any means of transport that requires them to be inside a cage (see Chapter 9). It is one of the components of the separation anxiety formula (see Section 5.2, p.111).

LOCAL APPLICATION

No known application.

Application to humans

KEY WORDS: Extreme anguish. Suffering and despair.

This temporary state is one of the most intense and painful of the Floral system. People in this state reach the limit of their mental, emotional and physical resistance and are helpless and defenceless against an unexpected obstacle or an apparently hopeless situation. This could include a separation, the death of a loved one or losing a job – the collapse of 'imaginary castles'. They think that they have wasted their life or changed their belief system and feel they have hit rock bottom. People in a Sweet

Chestnut state are immersed in the deepest darkness and unable to find a way out. This state plunges them into extreme existential angst, an interior void and profound despair. Sweet Chestnut's great suffering is caused by the refusal and resistance to accept that something significant but very painful has happened in their lives, whilst simultaneously repressing their feelings and most painful emotions. They are desperate, have hit rock bottom and feel their lives have no meaning. Sometimes the despair is so intense that they think about committing suicide.

4.31 Vervain (Verbena officinalis)

Those with fixed principles and ideas, which they are confident are right, and which they very rarely change.

They have a great wish to convert all around them to their own views of life.

They are strong of will and have much courage when they are convinced of those things that they wish to teach.

In illness they struggle on long after many would have given up their duties. (Bach 1936)

Application to animals

KEY WORDS: Enthusiasm (E.B.). Inflammation (R.O.). Excessive manifestation (TP).

ORAL APPLICATION

Vervain (excessive manifestation) is used to manage the internal tension and excitement experienced by hyperactive, restless, nervous, obsessive and stressed animals. It helps regulate every 'hyper' emotion. It is part of the formula for territorial, possessive and redirected aggressiveness (see Section 5.1.3, p.108).

It is also part of the formulas used to treat separation anxiety (see Section 5.2, p.111), stereotypic behaviour (see Section 5.7, p.120), canine hyperactivity disorder (see Section 5.9, p.123) and kennel cough (see p.225), and to lower the stress levels of animals that live in very small spaces and have no opportunity to run and burn off their excess energy.

It is an important remedy for animals that have not experienced a socialization period. Vervain enhances a puppy's exploratory capacities.

LOCAL APPLICATION

As a cream or Aloe Vera gel, and together with other remedies, Vervain (inflammation) is used to treat inflammation in any type of traumatism, abscesses, skin allergies, osteoarthritis, swollen lumps, inflammation of the anal glands, wounds, mastitis, stings, and so on. In eye-drop form it is part of the formula used to treat infectious and/or allergic conjunctivitis and inflammation of the third eyelid, and also in the formula for otitis (see Chapter 9).

Application to humans

> **KEY WORDS:** Excessive enthusiasm. Fanaticism and idealism.

Vervain people are very enthusiastic, idealistic, hyperactive, impulsive and intense, thus exhausting their energy striving for a better world or idea. They are considered to be the Robin Hoods of the Floral system, as they are extremely sensitive to injustices and they need to share their ideas and experiences with others to persuade them to follow the same path. Vervain people seek to transmit their enthusiasm and stir the spirits of others. Dragging people into their cause is the most important and urgent thing to them, and they become indignant when they do not understand why not everyone is joining their fight. This is when they despair and become unkind. Furthermore, Vervain people need others to connect immediately with their ideology. Their excess of enthusiasm often makes them fanatic people who tend to alienate others. Vervain people overexert themselves in everything they undertake (and they undertake a lot), which causes stress, tension and insomnia. As they are unable to relax they go beyond their physical limits. They put their life at stake to make the world a better place, or at least to improve conditions somewhere in the world. When they are not obeyed they react very badly, and this may even lead to episodes of aggressiveness and anger.

Vervain people focus on and undertake only those tasks they enjoy, becoming completely absorbed by them. Everything else becomes trivial and receives little of their attention.

4.32 Vine (Vitis vinifera)

Very capable people, certain of their own ability, confident of success.

Being so assured, they think that it would be for the benefit of others if they could be persuaded to do things as they themselves do, or as they are certain is right. Even in illness they will direct their attendants.

They may be of great value in emergency. (Bach 1936)

Application to animals

KEY WORDS: Domination (E.B.). Liquid causing pressure (R.O.). Territoriality.

ORAL APPLICATION

Vine (domination) is part of the formula for treating territorial, possessive and redirected aggressiveness (see Section 5.1.3, p.108). Together with other remedies it is used as a preventive treatment when the animal's owner is pregnant and is recommended to treat the animal throughout the owner's pregnancy and after childbirth (see Section 5.3, p.113).

LOCAL APPLICATION

As a cream or Aloe Vera gel, and together with other remedies, Vine (liquid causing pressure) is used locally to treat any condition that contains liquid (water, pus, etc.), whether it drains outwards or not. Examples include abscesses, swollen lumps, sores, anal glands containing liquid that has thickened or solidified, mastitis and otitis (see Chapter 9).

Application to humans

KEY WORDS: Dominant. Inflexible.

People in a Vine state dominate others. As they see it, their dictatorial attitudes have no negative effects because they are totally convinced they are doing the right thing; they do not doubt they have leadership qualities, that is, the ambition and ability to lead in order to 'help the rest'.

They are aggressive, ambitious, proud and arrogant. They may eagerly aspire to obtain power and can even be very cruel. They ignore others' opinions; they do not ask, they order. For them there is only one truth: their own. Because their intrinsic nature is to dominate, Vine people often do not understand or deal with the accusations they receive related to their power-mongering. They are also very manipulative and Machiavellian, attitudes that they use to thrive in the political, emotional or professional fields. When these 'arts' do not help them to achieve their purpose, they do not hesitate to frighten those around them and, if necessary, use verbal aggression. Vine people manipulate others coldly using their knowledge and intelligence to benefit themselves. They are therefore cold, rigid, inflexible and intolerant with whoever challenges their authority, always justifying these attitudes with 'I will not give in, I do it for your own good.' Furthermore, they demand blind obedience because they are convinced they are always right ('Because I say so! Period!'), and if necessary they will not hesitate to use domination and tyranny to achieve their aims.

However, when people in a Vine state are balanced, they are great educators, leaders and bosses. In emergency and crisis situations they have a global view and are able to save the situation thanks to their good perceptiveness and clarity of mind, and because they keep their cool.

4.33 Walnut (Juglans regia)

For those who have definite ideals and ambitions in life and are fulfilling them, but on rare occasions are tempted to be led away from their own ideas, aims and work by the enthusiasm, convictions or strong opinions of others.

The remedy gives constancy and protection from outside influences. (Bach 1936)

Application to animals

KEY WORDS: Adaptation (TP). Cut (TP).

ORAL APPLICATION

Walnut (adaptation) is the remedy used to facilitate an animal's adaptation to any change. At times it has to be used together with Holly as the latter deals with an animal's extreme sensitivity to a specific change, such as adoption, pseudopregnancy, owner's pregnancy, new life in an animal shelter or kennel, and so on.

Cats often require this remedy because they are very sensitive to change. Some see the arrival of a new baby, animal, or the owner's new partner as a 'dethronement'. Walnut will help them adapt better to these situations and inhibit any possible redirected aggressiveness (see Section 5.1.3, p.108).

Rock Water (resistance to change) and Chestnut Bud (learning process) together with Walnut (adaptation) are recommended for those animals that display a persistent behavioural problem.

Walnut is also part of the formula that helps animals with travel sickness (see Chapter 9, p.236), feline social aggressiveness (see Section 5.1.5, p.110) or maternal aggressiveness (see Section 5.1.2, p.107), those in heat (see Chapter 9, p.233), those with pseudocyesis (psychological pregnancy) (see Section 5.12, p.130), and those that defecate and urinate in inappropriate places (see Section 5.6, p.118). It is also one of the components of the formula for colds (see Chapter 9, p.231).

LOCAL APPLICATION

Walnut (cut) has proved effective as a blood-clotting agent in cuts, wounds, bites and other injuries that bleed, such as in the case of infected anal glands (see Case 7.4, p.198).

Application to humans

KEY WORDS: Protection and adaptation to changes and influences.

This remedy is used during periods of major changes in life, such as teething, puberty, pregnancy, menopause, divorce, moving house, change of profession, and so on. It helps the transition from the old to the new. It supports in making the necessary decisions for the vital change, not allowing outside influences to deviate us from those decisions or our path. Walnut enhances perseverance and constancy in what we have decided. It helps us connect with our intuition, allowing us to see the consequences of our ideas, aims and decisions, and find unconventional solutions that are far from the patterns imposed by family and society.

Walnut is also useful when trying to give up deep-rooted addictions or when breaking old bonds (habits, emotional ties, attitudes, etc.).

4.34 Water Violet (Hottonia plasters)

For those who in health or illness like to be alone. Very quiet people, who move about without noise, speak little, and then gently. Very independent, capable and self-reliant. Almost free of the opinions of others. They are aloof, leave people alone and go their own way. Often clever and talented. Their peace and calmness is a blessing to those around them. (Bach 1936)

Application to animals

KEY WORDS: Isolation.

ORAL APPLICATION

This remedy is of great help for cats or other animals that are prone to excessive isolation. Water Violet used together with Beech (intolerance) helps manage the animal's tendency to withdraw itself. A cat can spend many hours, even days, in an area called its 'isolation field'. When it does so not because it is stressed or sick, but because it is rejecting or avoiding social contact, the problem should be treated with Water Violet and Beech. Isolation fields are the areas where the animal withdraws and avoids contact with people and/or other animals. Most cats choose three isolation fields: these may be radiators, the owner's bed, inside a cupboard, and so on. Isolation fields serve as a refuge when something is difficult for them, and are usually located high up. In unsociable cats, the litter tray may be an isolation field.

LOCAL APPLICATION

In eye-drops (sterile saline solution) Water Violet is used to improve ocular dryness as, according to the work of Pablo Noriega (2006).

Application to humans

KEY WORDS: Pride and reservation.

Water Violet people have a feeling of superiority that, taken to the extreme, can make them cold, arrogant and condescending.

When in balance, they are polite, erudite and self-assured. They are often sought after because they give good advice and because they do not impose their views on others. This makes them good bosses and teachers.

Water Violet people do not like to dominate or be dominated. Neither do they like to interfere in the problems of others because they do not like others to interfere in theirs; in particular, they do not like their privacy to be invaded. For this reason, and because of their need to go unnoticed, they are located in Bach's category of loneliness where they feel quite comfortable.

Water Violet people have a tendency to get lost in their thoughts and keep their problems to themselves, never relying on others. They avoid conflicts, because they see them as beneath their dignity, and resolve their own problems alone. They do so first, because they are unable to seek help from anyone (this illustrates their sense of self-sufficiency) and second, because they are convinced that no one is capable of understanding their difficulties. They are selective in their relationships and need their time and solitude.

4.35 White Chestnut (Aesculus hippocastanum)

For those who cannot prevent thoughts, ideas, arguments which they do not desire from entering their minds. Usually at such times when the interest of the moment is not strong enough to keep the mind full.

Thoughts which worry and will remain, or if for a time thrown out, will return. They seem to circle round and round and cause mental torture.

The presence of such unpleasant thoughts drives out peace and interferes with being able to think only of the work or pleasure of the day. (Bach 1936)

Application to animals

KEY WORDS: Obsession (E.B.). Accelerated repetition (TP).

ORAL APPLICATION

White Chestnut (accelerated repetition) is the main remedy used to deal with stereotypic behaviours.[2] It is part of the formulas that treat separation anxiety (see Section 5.2, p.111); territorial, possessive and redirected aggressiveness (see Section 5.1.3, p.108); canine hyperactivity (see Section 5.9, p.123); and kennel cough (see p.225).

It is also used to treat restless and nervous animals and those with a fixation for attacking one particular animal. In general, White Chestnut helps animals with an active character, regardless of whether they do or do not show overexcitement.

LOCAL APPLICATION

No known application.

---

2   Stereotypic behaviour is a pattern of repetitive behaviour, carried out consistently and lacking function. The most common types in canines are chasing and mutilating the tail (tail-chasing); walking in circles (circling); self-licking injuries, usually in the area in front of the carpus (acral lick dermatitis); and constant barking. This may occur when the animal is deprived of social relationships with other animals, when it does not receive sufficient attention from the owners, or simply when it is bored and anxious.

Application to humans

KEY WORDS: Persistent thoughts. Tortuous internal dialogue.

White Chestnut helps those who have haunting and disturbing thoughts, ideas or images, or simply just repetitive ones which they can neither get rid of nor control. This exaggerated and repetitive mental activity can cause mental torment and fatigue, headache, tension in the forehead and behind the eyes, nervousness, internal agitation, insomnia and lack of concentration and attention. People in this state have a repetitive mental mechanism to avoid thinking about something they really should be thinking about (a relationship crisis, a frustrating job, a specific fear, the illness of a loved one, guilt, etc.). They therefore think about minor issues over and over without being able to find solutions, avoiding their real problems.

White Chestnut people abide by a mental pattern of obsession. Sometimes Cherry Plum and Scleranthus should be taken together with White Chestnut in order to reduce the obsessive tendencies.

People in a White Chestnut state take their mental confusion to bed with them and are unable to fall asleep. They lie restless, weighed down by the same thoughts, and even by images. Some manage to sleep but wake up in the middle of the night, victim of thoughts that they cannot keep away. Others have ended up being victims of an accident or being run over because they were distracted by continuous repetitive thoughts that kept them distant from reality.

4.36 Wild Oat (Bromus ramous)

Those who have ambitions to do something of prominence in life, who wish to have much experience, and enjoy all that which is possible for them, to take life to the full.

Their difficulty is to determine what occupation to follow; as although their ambitions are strong, they have no calling which appeals to them above all others.
This may cause delay and dissatisfaction. (Bach 1936)

Application to animals

Key words: None.

Oral application
No known application.

Local application
No known application.

Application to humans

Key words: Dissatisfaction. Doubts about the correct path in life.

Wild Oat helps people who have reached a crossroads in their life and are very doubtful of what way to go. They want to live life intensely but are not sure where to start. People in this state may do various different activities but find it very difficult to know which one corresponds to their mission in life. They are aware that life is passing by without them and thus feel frustrated and unfulfilled.

They may be ambitious, have a wide variety of talents and study for various university courses but often get bored and waste their talents due to the lack of a well-defined goal in their lives. This state is typical of those who after reaching a goal (finishing their studies, their children leaving home, etc.) then say: 'And now what do I do?'

The Wild Oat state corresponds to those moments in life when people, faced with a major change, lack the guidance to deal with the change and follow the right path. It is typical in those teenagers who, facing the many possibilities that life offers, cannot see which one they should follow and have difficulty making a commitment.

Wild Oat people are constantly searching because they have not yet found their place.

4.37 Wild Rose (Rosa canina)

Those who without apparently sufficient reason become resigned to all that happens, and just glide through life, take it as it is, without any effort to improve things and find some joy. They have surrendered to the struggle of life without complaint. (Bach 1936)

Application to animals

KEY WORDS: Apathy (E.B.).

ORAL APPLICATION

Wild Rose (apathy) is used as a secondary remedy for animals that remain in a corner without interacting with their environment. Sometimes they do not even want to eat or drink (some of these cases are the result of having been mistreated by their owners).

It is also used to treat apathetic dogs that manifest a lack of attention and motivation when faced with mental stimuli.

It is also important to treat the states underlying the Wild Rose animal's apathy, for example a Rock Rose (panic) state or a Star of Bethlehem (shock) state.

LOCAL APPLICATION

No known application.

Application to humans

KEY WORDS: Resignation and apathy.

Wild Rose is a state without horizons or prospects for the future. It is a state of absolute indifference where people have neither the motivation nor the energy to get out of the situation which they consider normal; they therefore accept the situation and give in without complaining and without suffering. They give up without regretting, surrendering a 'battle' in which they have not taken part.

Wild Rose people are those who are resigned to an unpleasant situation: an illness, a monotonous life or an unpleasant job. Change horrifies them. They are not miserable, and nor do they complain, but they are too apathetic to feel well, to change job or to enjoy simple pleasures.

4.38 Willow (Salix vitellina)

For those who have suffered adversity or misfortune and find these difficult to accept, without complaint or resentment, as they judge life much by the success which it brings.

They feel that they have not deserved so great a trial, that it was unjust, and they become embittered.

They often take less interest and are less active in those things of life which they had previously enjoyed. (Bach 1936)

Application to animals

KEY WORDS: Resentment (E.B.). Retention (TP).

Oral application

Initially there was no known relationship between Willow and the animal world until it was proven that a large number of cats that defecated in inappropriate places improved their anomalous behaviour when Willow was added to their formula.

Defecating in inappropriate places is one of the ways in which a cat expresses its dissatisfaction, for example if its owner has returned home later than usual. This phenomenon must not be confused with an animal that defecates in inappropriate places due to a temporary gastrointestinal problem (the vet will solve this problem), or separation anxiety in dogs where excretion in an inappropriate place is due to the anxiety itself.

Willow (resentment) should be complemented with other remedies, especially if the animal is in a state corresponding to Chicory (possessive), Heather (demanding attention), Holly (jealous) or Beech (intolerant).

Local application

No known application.

Application to humans

Key words: Resentment, bitterness and hardness of heart.

Willow people are those who feel resentment of others' luck, health, happiness or success. People in this state are grumpy, irritable, critical, moody, bitter, negative, stingy, envious and resentful killjoys, blaming everybody and enjoying complaining and transmitting sorrow to others. Sometimes the negativity of Willow does not become apparent until a conversation takes place and their repressed anger leads them to 'get stuck' in dispute. This is because Willow people are not satisfied with their balance of life and always find someone to blame for their bad luck (the doctors are to blame for their poor health, their parents' financial situation ruined their life, etc.).

Given their tendency to act the victim and display dissatisfaction when they are ill, they can appear unwilling to admit any improvement. Moreover, if their dreams, desires or ideals are not fulfilled, they express all their frustrations and disappointments by blaming family, friends, society, God or fate. Although they do not explode or become aggressive, they are constantly complaining, thereby poisoning their environment with their negativity, destructiveness and envy.

5

MOST COMMON
BEHAVIOURAL
PROBLEMS

This book is a practical help guide, in which solutions can be found for the most common behavioural problems in animals in order to improve their coexistence with and adaptation to the world around them (other animals, babies, children, their owners, their environment, etc.). However, it should never replace the work of vets, canine trainers, or behaviourists.

When an animal presents a behavioural problem, we must first take it to the vet in order to rule out the possibility that its behavioural changes may be rooted in a physical problem. In any therapy aimed to treat behavioural problems, we must always consider to what extent the owner or the environment is responsible for the animal's anomalous behaviour. In this respect, guidelines from an behaviourist or canine trainer are essential for teaching owners not to humanize their animals' feelings and to distinguish when the behaviour, although disturbing, is part of their intrinsic nature and when it is pathological. Therefore, close collaboration between vets, canine trainers and Bach Flower Therapists is essential to ensure that the correct solution to the animal's behavioural problem is found.

This chapter describes the most common behaviour problems in the canine and feline world, and their treatment with Bach Flowers. Although this part of the book refers mainly to cats and dogs, everything described below is applicable to all types of animals. Remember that the 38-Flower system discovered by Dr Bach is applicable to any living being, be it a human, animal or plant species.

In the following cases of aggressiveness, if the animal doesn't show any sign of improvement after two to three weeks of treating it with a Flower formula at a minimum frequency of five times per day, I recommend adding Chestnut Bud (if it wasn't included before) in order to boost the animal's learning capacity and response towards the situation which causes the anomalous behaviour. If the frequency of the treatment is fewer than five times per day, you will need to be more patient and wait for longer before changing the composition of the formula. Another option, again if it wasn't included in the formula, is to add Rock Water, the remedy responsible for making the subject overcome its resistance to change. Both Chestnut Bud and Rock Water could be added at the same time, depending on the therapist's criteria.

An obstacle often encountered by a Flower Therapist when treating problematic behaviours in animals is the difficulty of administering the remedies at the right frequency. Many people who administer the remedy to their animals don't have enough free time to comply with the recommended frequency for the treatment (i.e. a minimum of 4 drops, four times a day). Others forget a dose. This is the reason why we often recommend a frequency of four to five times per day, despite the fact that the problem to be treated requires a higher frequency – 4 drops, seven or eight times a day – especially at the beginning of the treatment. Even then, a frequency of four to five times per day may be difficult to keep to, as the majority of owners do not have enough free time. This means that sometimes the treatment takes longer to accomplish the desired results, whereas a higher frequency would solve the problem sooner. It is important to warn whoever is in charge of administering the treatment of this in advance, in order to avoid him or her abandoning it prematurely.

5.1 Aggressiveness

When facing a problem of aggressiveness, it is first advisable to go to a specialized professional (veterinarian, dog trainer, behaviourist) who will diagnose what type of aggressiveness the animal presents and the possible causes. Aggressiveness is a very complex behavioural problem that may have many different causes, and each one of them requires a different treatment.

Some animals present aggressive behaviour as a result of an organic or physiological problem. There are hormonal pathologies, such as hypothyroidism, intracranial tumours (if they affect the limbic system), hydrocephalus,[1] and epilepsy, that may cause aggressiveness in the animal. The animal that suffers from otitis may manifest secondary aggressiveness (see Section 5.1.4, p.109), an aggressiveness that has an organic cause.

In the cases of some dogs with aggressive behaviours it has been necessary to combine Flower Remedy treatment and canine training or therapy, with the help of a professional. In other cases, in either cats or dogs, it has also been necessary to treat the owners and/or the animals that live alongside the animal in question, in order to solve the problem more easily.

On other occasions, the aggressiveness between animals, or between an animal and a human, is generated when the other animal or the human doesn't know how to interpret the signals that the animal uses to communicate or establish relationships (this generates high levels of stress that cause fear-induced aggressiveness). With reference to this matter, we must highlight the great work carried out by Turid Rugaas; see her book *On Talking Terms with Dogs: Calming Signals* (Rugaas 1997).

Aggressiveness can take place between individuals of different species (interspecific aggressiveness), for example from a dog

---

1   Hydrocephalus is one of the most common growth alterations in dogs and starts to manifest between the fourth and sixth month of life. This condition involves an excessive accumulation of cerebrospinal fluid (the liquid that bathes the brain structures, cushioning these from impact with the skull).

towards a person, or between members of the same species, such as from a dog towards another dog (intraspecific aggressiveness).

The following are the most common types of aggressiveness that I have treated with Bach Flower Remedies.

5.1.1 Fear-induced aggressiveness

Fear-induced aggressiveness is usually directed towards any stimulus that creates fear or mistrust, including people, dogs, cats, other animals, and even objects. This uncomfortable situation, and not being able to escape from it, makes the animal react aggressively in order to defend itself and, depending on the dog, it may even bite, potentially causing serious injuries. The only thing the animal intends to do is ward off the fear-producing stimulus.

A dog that feels threatened will probably try to escape and, if unable to do so, will attack. Something similar may happen in the case of a frightened cat, but thanks to its agility and size the animal may be able to escape and not generate aggression, thus avoiding confrontation with the person or animal that has caused its fear. The situation becomes dangerous if the cat does not find a way out; pain and fear are very strong and important stimuli in triggering feline aggressiveness. This type of aggressiveness is the most common cause of bites and scratches from cats.

Fear-induced aggressiveness may be related to poor socialization or lack of imprinting (see Section 5.10, p.124, and Section 5.13, p.132). To address this type of aggressiveness you need to consider remedies that manage fear and/or panic and the after effects arising from traumatic stress in an animal that feels threatened. You should also consider remedies that manage aggressiveness due to mistrust, rejection of whatever frightens it or hysteria towards the stimulus that it experiences as a threat.

The following remedies should be considered for this type of aggressiveness:

Rock Rose (terror, panic) + Star of Bethlehem (trauma, shock) + Beech (intolerance, rejection) + Cherry Plum (lack of control, hysteria) + Holly (mistrust).

This formula should be administered at a rate of 4 drops, four to six or more times per day, depending on the level of aggressiveness of the animal, in direct application whenever possible.

5.1.2 Maternal aggressiveness

Female dogs develop this aggressiveness towards people and/or animals that get close to their puppies when they are a few days old. In general, this behaviour disappears one month after giving birth.

For this type of aggressiveness, a preventive treatment with Bach Flowers from approximately one month before to one month after delivery is recommended to regulate the hormone influence characteristic of this maternal period.

Any female who has just given birth protects her young. It is part of her maternal instinct. The problem arises when the female becomes afraid and overly mistrustful, not trusting those who approach what she feels is her own private property. She usually rejects visitors by establishing boundaries with signals of aggressiveness, and in some cases attacks them due to an out-of-control impulse that has the protection of her young as its main objective.

The following Bach Flowers should be considered for maternal aggressiveness:

Beech (intolerance and rejection) + Cherry Plum (lack of control, hysteria) + Chicory (possessiveness) + Holly (mistrust) + Rock Rose (panic) + Walnut (adaptation).

This formula should be administered at a rate of 4 drops, four to six or more times per day depending on the level of aggressiveness in the animal, in direct application whenever possible.

5.1.3 Territorial, possessive and redirected aggressiveness

Territorial aggressiveness occurs when an intruder (human or animal) appears in the territory (house, garden, car, etc.) that the dog considers its own.

Cats also defend their territory. This behaviour is normal but becomes a behavioural problem when two or more cats live in the same house and direct the aggression at each other.

Possessive aggressiveness is induced when an animal tries to defend its food, toys or any other valuable objects (resource guarding), or tries to protect a person.

Redirected aggressiveness occurs when the dog or cat cannot attack the person or animal that generates a negative stimulus and instead attacks another more accessible person or animal (see Case 6.1.2, p.140, and Case 6.1.4, p.144).

These three types of aggressiveness correspond to the natural behaviour of dogs, as they allow them to regulate relationships between members of the pack and ensure their survival. You should therefore consider remedies that treat excessive territoriality or competitive dominance and extreme possessiveness towards people, food or objects. Remedies that manage mistrust of and low tolerance towards anyone who enters the animal's territory and those that regulate excitement and lack of control due to this external stimulus should also be considered.

The following Bach Flowers should be considered for these three types of aggressiveness:

> Beech (intolerance and rejection) + Cherry Plum (lack of control, hysteria) + Chicory (possessiveness) + Holly (mistrust) + Vine (domination, territoriality) + Vervain (overexcitement) + White Chestnut (repetition, obsession).

This formula should be administered at a rate of 4 drops, four to six or more times per day depending on the level of aggressiveness of the animal, in direct application whenever possible.

In the case of cats, we usually have to add Willow (resentment) and Walnut (adaptation) to their formula. Cats are not good at accepting changes and may sometimes manifest their dissatisfaction by scratching, hissing in disagreement or defecating and urinating in inappropriate places. This can happen when the owner changes partner, when a visitor prevents the owner from paying the cat enough attention or when the owner is away too much.

5.1.4 Secondary aggressiveness

This type of aggressiveness is a response to pain or illness. It usually occurs when we touch an area where the animal feels pain. For example, a dog with acute otitis may show aggressive behaviour if you touch its ear when you stroke its head.

Since this is a sporadic aggressive situation, it is important to treat the animal with Rescue Remedy as that will stabilize it rapidly in any specific stressful situation (e.g. treating and dressing wounds that cause the animal pain). It may also be helpful to add Cherry Plum and Star of Bethlehem, despite these already being included in the Rescue Remedy formula, because this aggressiveness stems from a physical traumatism and the animal usually responds in an uncontrolled manner to pain that is sensitive to touch.

The following Bach Flowers should be selected for secondary aggressiveness:

> Rescue Remedy (emergency) + Cherry Plum (lack of control, hysteria) + Elm (pain sensitive to touch) + Star of Bethlehem (shock).

If the animal is of a fearful nature or it is scared as a result of the physical trauma it has experienced (e.g. being run over, a contusion, a bite from another animal, etc.), add Rock Rose (panic) to the formula above.

This formula should be administered at a rate of 4 drops, four to six or more times per day depending on the level of aggressiveness of the animal, in direct application whenever possible.

5.1.5 Feline social aggression

Feline social aggression is the type of aggressiveness that an adult cat directs towards a kitten that has recently joined its home. This behaviour originates from the fact that two felines don't feel they belong to the same species if they are not in the same stage of development. This is what happens between a kitten and an adult, and this is a major problem if the two have to coexist in the same space.

A kitten has a gregarious social behaviour pattern until it reaches 8–12 months – the age at which kittens usually leave their mother to find their own territory and adopt the unsocial behaviour typical of adult male cats. When a kitten approaches an adult cat, the latter may attack the kitten because, according to the adult's point of view, the kitten did not respect the basic feline laws of social, personal and critical distances.

Beech is the typological Bach Flower for cats and is also common to certain types of aggressiveness. It is important that the adult cat's intolerance and rejection towards kittens be managed with Beech, and its aggressiveness due to jealousy towards kittens with Holly.

Cats have difficulty tolerating changes. Walnut and Rock Water can help a cat deal with the introduction of a kitten. Remember too that Chestnut Bud will help the cat to assimilate better the information from the other remedies contained in the formula.

The following Bach Flowers are used for treating feline social aggression:

> Beech (intolerance) + Holly (jealousy) + Chestnut Bud (learning process) + Rock Water (resistance to change) + Walnut (adaptation).

These five remedies are the basic ones for this type of aggressiveness, but if the adult cat is very territorial and possessive, also add Chicory and/or Vine. If, with the arrival of a kitten, the adult adopts inappropriate toilet habits (see Section 5.6, 'Defecation and urination in inappropriate places', p.118), add Willow to its formula.

This formula should be administered at a rate of 4 drops, four to six or more times per day depending on the level of aggressiveness of the animal, in direct application whenever possible.

5.2 Separation anxiety

This is a behavioural disorder characterized by signs of distress that occur when the dog is alone or separated from its owner. The signs to be observed include destruction of furniture, clothes, walls, doors and household items (destructive behaviour); never-ending barking; inappropriate excretion (anxiety encourages the sphincters to open); and recurrent whining.

The animal's behaviour is often different when it is accompanied from when it is alone. This behavioural problem, together with aggressiveness, is one of the main causes of animal abandonment.

The factors that trigger this type of anxiety are diverse. The most important ones include:

- Animals that are very affectionate and dependent on the owner. Often this behaviour is induced by the owner's emotional needs.

- The type of bond between the dog and its owner.

- Returning to a state of solitude after a long period of coexistence with the owner, such as a weekend, trip, summer holiday, and so on.

- Recent adoptions. When moving from a shelter to a home, some animals experience anxiety for a few days. In the shelter they coexist with other animals and are never alone, whereas at home they are not always accompanied.

When treating separation anxiety in a dog, guidelines from a canine trainer or behaviourist are important. First, they are aimed at changing certain habits in the animal, and second, and sometimes more important, they help the owners to understand that their pet is not human and should not be treated as such if they don't want to perpetuate the separation anxiety pathology.

It is also necessary to treat the dogs, and if possible their owners, with Flower Remedies, thus reinforcing the work done by the canine education professional.

Bach Flowers selected to treat separation anxiety

The main aims of the Flower formula that treats separation anxiety are to lower the anxiety and stress level that the animal suffers when feeling lonely and deal with the physical manifestations that arise from this, such as hyperventilation, accelerating heartbeat, and so on. It is also necessary to regulate their need to be always in someone's company and their excessive demands for attention.

My experience in treating separation anxiety has led me to include a remedy to treat phobia in the formula. Behind the anxiety lies an important component of phobia (fear) that is not always covered by the other remedies.

> Agrimony (anxiety) + Impatiens (acceleration) + Sweet Chestnut (extreme anguish) + Vervain (over excitation, hyperactivity) + White Chestnut (repetition) + Chicory (possessiveness) + Heather (demanding attention) + Rock Rose (panic).

In animals with high stress levels you should administer Rescue Remedy (emergency) instead of Impatiens. This formula should be administered at a rate of 4 drops, four to six times per day depending on the animal's anxiety levels, in direct application whenever possible. If after two to three weeks of treatment, at a minimum rate of six times per day, the animal's behavioural problem persists, we recommend adding Rock Water (resistance to change) and Chestnut Bud (learning process) to the formula, instead of Sweet Chestnut. If the frequency of administration is low, you should wait longer for results.

The canine trainer and Flower Therapist Antonio Paramio discovered that there are certain unbalanced behaviours in animals and the humans who live with them that are not the result of an adaptation problem (Walnut). Rather, these are problems of resistance to change (Rock Water) that stem from well-established behavioural patterns due to the age and experience of the animal. As Antonio Paramio (2009) says himself, if we add to this the fact that dogs are quite obsessive-compulsive in their behaviours and routines, the need to include this remedy is clear. All treatment is aimed at achieving behavioural change and, to accomplish this, it is necessary to eliminate the resistance to change.

In a talk he gave at the Active Fridays, one of the free activities organized by SEDIBAC (Society for the Study and Promotion of Bach Flower Remedies in Catalonia), Ricardo Orozco (2007) suggested the idea of administering Centaury (subjugation and dependency) to treat this type of conduct. Some people adopt a dog into their home to fulfil their own emotional needs, inducing in the animal an absolute dependence on them. Over time, this excessive dependence can become a behavioural problem. At present, Centaury is a remedy that is still under study in the treatment of this disorder.

5.3 Jealousy: A baby's arrival

The owner's pregnancy

If the animal has a behavioural problem before its owner's pregnancy it must be corrected with the help of a professional (canine trainer or behaviourist). Any problem, however small it may seem, could get worse after the baby's birth.

Changes in the animal's routines (walking times, restricted rooms, etc.) must be introduced before the baby arrives. It is recommended that the dog be engaged in the changes of furniture arrangement, allowing it to smell all the baby's new furniture, and some of its clothing and equipment (its cot, pushchair, etc.). As treatment with the new behavioural guidelines progresses and the animal's relationship with the owners improves, it will be time to start practising with a doll wrapped in baby clothes, perfumed with a product that will be used on the baby (e.g. a powder), and simulating entering and exiting the home cradling the 'baby' in their arms. The 'baby' is shown to the animal so it can smell it, and it will be rewarded affectionately for not jumping up at the 'baby'. It is also suggested that the dog is walked with the pushchair before the baby is born so that it starts to associate going for a walk with the pushchair as something pleasant.

The Bach Flower Remedy treatment has to help the animal cope with jealousy, rejection and adaptation to the situation that is to come and foster the animal's learning ability and assimilation of its new situation.

The following remedies should be considered when preparing an animal for the arrival of a baby:

> Beech (intolerance, rejection) + Chicory (possessiveness) + Heather (demanding attention) + Holly (jealousy) + Vine (territoriality) + Chestnut Bud (learning process) + Rock Water (resistance to change) + Walnut (adaptation).

This formula should be administered at a rate of 4 drops, four to six or more times per day, in direct application whenever possible. It is advisable to continue with the treatment after the baby is born in order to help the animal to deal better with living with it.

The arrival of a baby

The arrival of a baby usually consumes much of our time. When we have spare time and we are calm, for example when the baby is sleeping, we can use it to play with and pay more attention to our dog or cat, thus encouraging the animal not to feel so rejected. It is also important to positively reinforce the animal in front of the baby, caressing it, giving it small rewards or simply playing with it, and to support this with the Flower formula mentioned above, at a rate of 4 drops, a minimum of four times a day, in direct application if possible.

Add Willow to the formula instead of Chicory for a cat. Cats are likely to express dissatisfaction with the arrival of a new animal or baby in the family. Remember that they find it hard to adapt to change.

As time goes by, and when the baby grows and becomes a child, it will seek contact with the animal in order to play with it. The purpose and responsibility of parents is to teach their children that animals are not toys and that when they pull its ears, fur or tail the animal feels pain or stress and may respond with aggressiveness against these entirely negative stimuli. An animal will react much more positively to calm approaches and stroking.

5.4 Coprophagia

Coprophagia involves the ingestion of faeces by the animal, either its own or those of other animals or people. It is common in dogs and rarely occurs in cats.

In many cases this is due to a normal behaviour in the canine species. For example, female dogs eat faeces and urine from their puppies. There are adult dogs that eat the faeces of people or other animal species because of the high concentration of undigested proteins they contain. Thus coprophagia is not always a pathological behaviour, but rather a normal and ecological use of a food resource that is rich in protein and micronutrients, or it may simply reflect a vestigial instinct. However, some animals seek nutrients or micronutrients in the stools because they are lacking in vitamins and minerals, and this must be treated by a vet.

Sometimes an animal's coprophagia may have to do with the number of times it is fed each day; if it is fed only once, it is possible that it will spend the rest of the day trying to make up for the absence of food through this unpleasant behaviour. The problem may be solved by feeding it twice a day.

Before treating this disorder with Flower Remedies, it is essential to go to a vet in order to rule out the possibility that the animal's coprophagia is present due to a nutritional aetiology; digestive assimilation disorders such as pancreatitis; malabsorption syndrome; pancreatic insufficiency; intestinal infections; or an excess of fatty foods.

There are three kinds of coprophagia. Autocoprophagia occurs when the animal eats its own excrement; intraspecific coprophagia occurs when the animal ingests the faecal material of an animal that belongs to the same species; and interspecific coprophagia happens when the animal eats the faeces of an animal belonging to another species.

An animal that eats its own faeces will not normally cause itself any physical harm, but if it eats the faeces of other animals it could catch intestinal parasites or a viral disease such as hepatitis and parvovirus, or even toxoplasmosis if the faeces come from a cat infected with the *Toxoplasma gondii* parasite.

An animal may behave in this way due to boredom or having learned it from another animal close to it. Sometimes this behaviour begins when the animal sees its owner pick up stools every time it goes for a walk and the dog imitates this by picking one up with its mouth and eating it. A dog that starts a coprophagic behaviour may discover that it likes the taste, especially if the faeces are from a cat.

The Flower procedure for treating coprophagia essentially has to cover aspects of anxiety, boredom and attention seeking. The following Bach Flowers should be considered for dealing with this behavioural disorder:

Agrimony (anxiety) + Heather (demanding attention) + Impatiens (anxiety) + Rescue Remedy (calming effect).

This formula should be administered at a rate of 4 drops, four to six or more times per day depending on the level of anxiety of the animal, in direct application whenever possible.

5.5 Depression/sadness

An animal's sadness may be caused by a recent traumatic experience (e.g. the death of its owner or another animal that lived with it, being abandoned, etc.). Depression, however, is often related to a problem in its familiar environment. Often its owners do not pay it enough attention, they exclude it from family activities or it is left alone for long periods. This can cause boredom and apathy. Moreover, depression is caused by a lack of external stimuli such as games, petting and company, and in some cases by stress.

The Bach Flower Therapy treatment must address some of the various manifestations of a depressive syndrome (apathy, sadness, melancholy, etc.) depending in each case on what is being expressed by the animal that has to be treated. It is also important to consider and treat the cause that has led the animal to fall into a depression/depressive state.

Mustard (sadness), Honeysuckle (melancholy), Star of Bethlehem (trauma), Walnut (adaptation) and Gorse (giving up) are the remedies used to treat a dog that is sad because its owner has died. Some dogs spend long periods of time lying on the floor by the front door of the house, waiting for their owner to return. In rural areas there have been cases where the dog has spent hours lying in the entrance to the cemetery or place its owner was buried, without showing any interest in moving from the spot. These five remedies are also suitable for treating an animal that expresses sadness at the temporary or permanent absence of another animal that lived with it. If the animal also manifests a lack of energy, consider adding Olive (exhaustion) to the remedies mentioned above.

Also consider Rock Rose (panic) for the animal that, after losing its 'housemate', does not want to go outside for walks, or even to do its physiological necessities. This sometimes happens when the animal that lived with it did not return after leaving home one day (if it was put down due to an illness or old age, or if it was 'relocated' to another home – see Case 6.11.9, p.184).

In the case of an animal that manifests sadness, the basic Bach Flowers you should consider are:

> Gorse (giving up) + Mustard (sadness) + Star of Bethlehem (shock) + Walnut (adaptation) + remedies that consider the cause of its sadness (fear, death of a loved one, abandonment, etc.) + remedies to deal with other manifestations of its depressive state (apathy, exhaustion, melancholy).

This formula should be administered at a rate of 4 drops, four to six or more times per day depending on the case to be treated, in direct application whenever possible.

5.6 Defecation and urination in inappropriate places

Excretion in inappropriate places by both dogs and cats is a common reason for consultation. This disorder could be the result of some very different causes.

First, inappropriate excretion by felines and canines may be the manifestation of an organic disease, such as cystitis due to urinary crystals, stress or infection; joint pain (osteoarthritis or arthritis); or neurological deficiencies.

Second, in felines it can be caused by problems as simple as not having the litter box clean or having it in a place that the cat does not like, for example beside its food or water bowl or near to noisy household electrical appliances. Another cause can be that they are marking out their territory, in which case castration is often the solution. In 80–90 per cent of cases, inappropriate excretion is solved in this way, although there are some exceptional cases of cats that take months to correct this disorder.

Third, inappropriate excretion may the animal's way of manifesting that there is a stressful situation in its environment.

If an animal shows inappropriate excretion behaviour, you must first take it to the vet for examination and rule out any physical pathology that could justify its anomalous behaviour. For cats we must take into account the 'domestic' aspects mentioned above.

Finally, if there is neither an organic nor a domestic cause to explain the inappropriate excretion, we recommend treating it with Bach Flowers.

Cats have a hard time tolerating changes. They may urinate on their owner's bed or clothes when there is a house move or a change in partner, or simply when visitors prevent their owner from paying them enough attention. Beech (intolerance), Heather (demanding attention), Rock Water (resistance to change) and Walnut (adaptation) will be of great help in such situations. If the cat is of a possessive nature, also consider Chicory. If it is very territorial, consider Vine.

If the inappropriate excretion behaviour is due to the owner's pregnancy (some cats hiss as well as urinating on clothes) or due to the arrival of a new animal to the house, add Holly (jealousy). It is advisable to continue treatment after the owner gives birth so that the animal can deal better with the arrival of the baby.

A cat may also excrete in inappropriate places when it spends many hours alone at home. In this case the same remedies as in the previous cases should be considered.

In many cats that I have treated with this behavioural problem, their disorder has not been fully resolved until the remedy Willow (resentment) was added to the formula, as the cat may be using this inappropriate behaviour to express resentment at a change in its environment.

It has been proved that certain medications, including anxiolytics, reduce this type of behaviour, which suggests that they must be influenced by states of anxiety or stress.

To treat inappropriate excretion behaviour you should consider the following Bach Flowers:

Beech (intolerance) + Chicory (possessiveness) + Heather (demanding attention) + Holly (anger) + Willow (resentment) + Walnut (adaptation).

This formula should be administered at a rate of 4 drops, four to six or more times per day depending on the case to be treated, in direct application whenever possible, until the problem has been totally solved.

This problem may also occur in separation anxiety, mentioned previously (see p.111). In this case inappropriate excretion is due to the anxiety itself. This problem also arises in animals that have recently suffered a situation of great stress.

Small urinations by a dominant male dog are regarded as a sign that he is marking his territory. Although this behaviour is very annoying for the owners, we have not considered its treatment with Bach Flower Remedies because it is a very rare behaviour.

5.7 Stereotypic behaviour

Stereotypic behaviour is a pattern of repetitive, invariable behaviour that has no function. This can happen when the animal is deprived of social interaction with other animals, when it doesn't receive enough attention from its owners, or simply when it is bored and anxious.

The most common stereotypic behaviours in the canine world are chasing and mutilating the tail (tail-chasing), walking in circles (circling), skin damage due to licking, usually in the lower portion of the leg (acral lick dermatitis), and constant barking.

Flower treatment aiming to help an animal in this situation should consider the repetitive aspect involved in the specific stereotypic behaviour, as well as the causes that trigger it, especially attention-seeking and anxiety.

Listed below are the remedies that should be considered in the treatment of stereotypic behaviours:

> Agrimony (anxiety) + Heather (demanding attention) + Impatiens (acceleration) + Vervain (overexcitement) + White Chestnut (accelerated repetition) + Rescue Remedy (calming effect).

This formula should be administered at a rate of 4 drops, four to six or more times per day depending on the case to be treated, in direct application whenever possible.

5.8 Stress

Acute stress is an animal's response to danger. In this situation, the brain triggers the secretion of a series of steroid hormones such as adrenalin and cortisol, which prepare a dog's muscles to act vigorously, lower its reaction threshold and inhibit its rational functions. Thus the animal's body prepares to flee or fight. This reaction is essential in threatening situations, but is a problem if repeated on a daily basis. Chronic stress occurs when an animal experiences a threatening situation continuously and the substances involved in the body's response to that danger, by acting continuously, cause side effects in the animal due to excess cortisol in its organism. Consequently, the animal's body is motionless and it experiences a low resistance to pain and a state of lethargy. Canine depressions are frequently associated with chronic stress.

The Flower treatment for an animal that has experienced a specific situation of acute stress (e.g. being run over by a car without significant physical consequences, a fight with another animal, a fall or a contusion, a loud noise, etc.) should include those remedies that help the animal deal with the post-traumatic panic after effects, and those that regulate its level of excitement.

In most cases combining Rock Rose (panic) + Star of Bethlehem (shock) will be enough to restore the balance of the animal's nervous system when it has been affected by the experience of a stressful situation, and Vervain (overexcitement) + White Chestnut (acceleration, repetition) to deal with the hyperactivity that the stress-triggering situation has caused in the animal and which activates its fight-or-flight response. If the animal is very nervous and restless, Rescue Remedy can be added to the four remedies mentioned above; 4 drops, four times per day for two to three days, will be enough for the animal to return to its normal emotional state.

It is very important, and I would say essential, to treat every animal that has suffered a specific stressful situation with Flower Remedies. This is not because they are unable to restore their internal balance by themselves – only two or three days are needed – but because usually when an animal suffers an external stress-triggering stimulus (an attack by another dog, a contusion, etc.) before it can recover calmly by itself, it receives a second external stimulus: its owners will usually go running to its aid to console it, thereby sending out a vibration of worry and sometimes fear that the animal interprets as 'I am still in danger.' The animal continues expressing fear (howling, running away, etc.) way beyond the incident and suffers an emotional breakdown. So, what could have been a minor incident becomes a Rock Rose + Star of Bethlehem trauma. In some cases, an untreated animal will find it hard to recover from the trauma if its owners take it for walks, as it will be frightened and alert to the possibility of another attack by another dog. These animals are very likely to suffer from chronic stress.

The Flower treatment for an animal with chronic stress, in addition to rebalancing its nervous system, should take into consideration how the stress is shown. Some stressed animals experience emotions of fear. The remedies Rock Rose (panic) and Star of Bethlehem (shock, trauma) will help them manage the post-traumatic panic after effects. Some animals also hyperventilate due to the energy loss involved in living almost permanently on alert, and for them the Sweet Chestnut remedy (extreme anguish) will be of great help. Other animals become lethargic and need Clematis. Others become aggressive (see Section 5.1, p.105), or develop anxiety disorders (see Section 5.2, p.111) or problems of defecation and urination in inappropriate places (see Section 5.6, p.118).

A state of stress maintained for a long period of time causes side effects for the animal due to the excess of cortisol in its system. Olive will provide energy to the adrenal glands, which are responsible for producing cortisol. Therefore, this remedy is of great importance in the treatment of chronic stress, regardless of how the animal manifests it.

The treatment of an animal with this type of stress should last at least three months at a rate of 4 drops, four to six or more times per day, depending on the animal's stress level.

5.9 Canine hyperactivity disorder

Canine hyperactivity disorder can be observed in the early stages of the dog's development. This is the case of the puppy that, having an 'unlimited curiosity', investigates and chews everything within its reach. In short, it is discovering the world (smells, tastes, textures) and plays, runs, etc. Animals whose owners do not always use the same commands or do not use positive reinforcement, as well as those animals that exercise excessively, such as running and chasing the ball too much, are also at risk of suffering from canine hyperactivity.

The manifestations most commonly observed in acute canine hyperactivity disorder are: excessive nervous energy, fast heartbeat, increased breathing rate, attention deficit, salivation, constant movements and relentless barking. All these manifestations are symptoms associated with stress.

The high levels of overexcitement involved in canine hyperactivity can be treated with Vervain (overexcitement) and White Chestnut (accelerated repetition). The acceleration and anxiety present in most cases are treated with Impatiens (acceleration) and Agrimony (anxiety). In the most severe cases it is also recommended that Rescue Remedy (emergency) be added to the formula in order to stabilize the animal more quickly.

The Bach Flowers that must be considered in the treatment of canine hyperactivity disorder are as follows:

Rescue Remedy (emergency) + Agrimony (anxiety) + Impatiens (acceleration) + Vervain (overexcitement) + White Chestnut (accelerated repetition).

This formula will be administered at a rate of 4 drops, four to six or more times per day depending on the case to be treated, in direct application whenever possible.

It is not easy to administer the remedies directly into the mouth of some hyperactive animals; they move around a lot and some may even respond aggressively. In these cases you should administer the formula indirectly, despite the fact that this is not as effective as direct application.

5.10 Canine and feline filial imprinting

Imprinting is a biological learning process through which the offspring identify themselves with the adults of their own species. Observing and imitating the adults, they learn the various methods of survival, such as finding food and shelter, and models of defence, attack (learnt through play), coexistence, mating, and so on. In dogs and cats this process occurs in a period ranging from birth to three months of age.

A young animal that does not receive this essential imprinting will not learn from its mother the codes and signs it will need as an adult to interpret correctly the language and movements of other animals of the same species. This inability to interpret another animal of the same species correctly may lead to a negative reaction, including even aggressiveness or fear.

Whenever possible it is of the utmost importance to keep the young animal with its mother for at least the first four months of its life.

This process is treated with the same formulas as lack of socialization (see Section 5.13, p.132).

5.11 Fear and panic (phobia)

5.11.1 Noise-induced: parties and fireworks, storms, etc.

This is the fear and/or traumatic panic experienced by an animal as a result of an external loud noise that causes it great stress. The panic is repeated each time the animal is subject to the same or a similar noise. It is therefore recommended, and I would say essential, that the animal that has suffered this type of shock-trauma should receive preventive treatment whenever there is a celebration accompanied by fireworks in the town or city where it lives. It is enough to begin treatment a week in advance at a rate of 4 drops, four to six times per day. During the day before and the day of the celebration the formula should be administered at high frequency, every five minutes if the animal needs it and the owner's timetable allows it. Finally, the treatment should be maintained for two to three days after the stressful situation has come to an end.

The following Bach Flowers treat noise-induced fear and traumatic panic:

> Rock Rose (panic) + Star of Bethlehem (trauma, shock) + Sweet Chestnut (extreme anguish) + Rescue Remedy (emergency).

Administer the formula in direct application.

There are animals which, when confronted with a loud noise, and in addition to expressing a phobia (approaching the owner seeking protection, not wanting to go outside, etc.), start to get very nervous and anxious, experiencing a significant stress level. In these cases Vervain (overexcitement) and/or White Chestnut (repetition) and/or Impatiens (acceleration) should be added to its formula; choose one or more of these remedies depending on the animal's stress level.

5.11.2 Stress-related urine infections (feline idiopathic cystitis)

It is believed that cats with idiopathic cystitis may have a lower quantity of glycosaminoglycans in their bladder mucosa, a situation that predisposes them to be irritated by the action of the substances that are dissolved in the urine. In addition, it appears that any stress cats suffer, which may be caused by any change in their familiar environment, also increases the risk of a stress-related condition, such as a urine infection.

Any stressful situation (see Section 5.8, p.121) triggers off the sympathetic nervous system and hence the adrenal glands that cause an immediate secretion of cortisol. If this situation persists for a long period of time, on a continuous basis, it may produce a dysfunction of these glands, affecting the animal's emotional and immune system.

In this situation, the factors that trigger stress in the animal have to be taken into consideration when applying Bach Flowers. These usually include a traumatic change experienced with fear and/or panic that the animal is unable to adapt to or overcome. This causes inflammation and a subsequent infection of the lining of the bladder as well as inducing a state of exhaustion in the animal. You must therefore take into consideration the following Bach Flowers:

> Crab Apple (cleanse) + Olive (exhaustion) + Rock Rose (panic) + Star of Bethlehem (shock) + Walnut (adaptation).

This formula should be administered at a rate of 4 drops, four times per day, together with the treatment prescribed by the vet.

5.11.3 Due to abandonment and mistreatment

An animal that has been mistreated and/or abandoned will suffer from constant fear and traumatic panic situations that leave clear after effects on its emotional and physical state. When treating it you must therefore consider remedies that deal with the residues of post-traumatic fear and panic, as well as the low physical and emotional tone of the animal that has been under a permanent state of stress.

These animals, once adopted, continue to live in panic, even if they have a home and a family that cares for them. Moreover, if they are not treated they have a hard time trusting people; even when a familiar person approaches to pet them, they hide, seeking protection, or adopt a posture that indicates fear.

It is recommended that the animal that has been mistreated and/or abandoned be treated with the following Bach Flowers:

Rock Rose (panic) + Star of Bethlehem (shock, trauma) + Sweet Chestnut (extreme anguish) + Gorse (giving up) + Olive (exhaustion) + Walnut (adaptation).

This formula should be administered at first at a rate of 4 drops, four to six times a day in direct application for at least one month. The rate should then be 4 drops, four times a day for at least five more months.

In cases of this problem that have been treated, it has been proved that animals most often need a minimum of six months' treatment to begin to trust the people around them again. After being treated for two to three weeks with the above formula, many of the animals that initially manifested fear began to express their true nature or way of being that was concealed under the layer of traumatic panic. Some turned out to be possessive, and so Chicory needed to be added to the formula. Others were very attention-seeking, so Heather was added. Others were very territorial and required the Vine remedy. Others showed signs of aggressiveness, so Holly, Beech and Cherry Plum were added. Finally, others showed that beneath the panic resulting from mistreatment and/or abandonment, they already had a fearful nature. In all of these cases the formula mentioned above (plus the remedies required in each case) was administered for at least six months.

5.11.4 Due to the animal's intrinsic nature

Rock Rose is the main remedy used to treat an animal of a fearful nature. There are dogs of a Rock Rose nature that approach or hide behind their owner for protection even though they are not experiencing an imminent danger. Find out whether these animals were found on the street and may have experienced a situation of mistreatment before being abandoned.

In animals of this character type that have experienced situations of sustained stress, it is recommended that the action of Rock Rose be reinforced with the Star of Bethlehem remedy. It is also advised that Olive be administered in order to treat the exhaustion that the chronic stress has caused.

The Bach Flowers selected for this type of animal are as follows:

Rock Rose (panic) + Olive (exhaustion) + Star of Bethlehem
(if the animal has been mistreated, abandoned or run over).

This formula should be administered in direct application at a rate of 4 drops, four times per day for a three to six-month period.

Animals that show no signs of improvement after a month of treatment with the formula mentioned above will also need Chestnut Bud (learning process) and Rock Water (resistance to change) in their formula.

5.11.5 The preoperative and postoperative periods/visits to the veterinarian

Some animals get stressed when they have to go to the vet. Some even show signs of stress every time they pass near the door of the vet's surgery.

To help an animal that gets stressed in this situation, we recommend treating it with Flower Remedies one week before its visit to the vet. The same applies when the animal has to undergo surgery and during the postoperative period.

In these cases, the aspects of traumatic fear and panic experienced by the animal in a stressful situation, as well as the resulting anguish and the animal's lack of adaptation to that situation, must be considered in order to apply the correct formula. We must also take into account the exhaustion that the animal suffers when experiencing great stress.

The Bach Flowers that should be selected in these situations are as follows:

> Rescue Remedy (emergency) + Rock Rose (panic) + Star of Bethlehem (shock, trauma) + Sweet Chestnut (extreme anguish) + Walnut (adaptation).

This formula should be administered at a rate of 4 drops, four times per day in direct application, five days before the visit to the vet or an operation. The day before the stressful situation, add Olive to the formula, at a rate of 4 drops, eight to ten times per day. On the day of the vet visit or operation, apply the formula at a high frequency, 4 drops every half hour, and maintain this treatment for three more days at a frequency of four times per day.

People who do not have the complete set of Bach Flowers with which to develop their own formulas, and therefore must buy them at a pharmacy or a specialized store, can initially buy a formula that includes the above remedies plus Olive.

5.11.6 Travel

It is advisable to get a dog used to travelling by car from when it is a puppy. However, if the dog is already an adult and is stressed by travelling, we recommend treating it with Flower Remedies. Most animals affected by travelling hyperventilate and some even vomit.

If a long journey is planned, it is recommended that you carry out a preventive treatment one week before starting the trip, at a rate of 4 drops, four times per day by direct application, and on the day of the trip administer 4 drops every half hour. If the journey is by car, we recommend stopping every two hours and walking the dog for a few minutes, at the same time administering 4 drops of the formula. If the trip is by another means of transport that doesn't allow you to stop the formula can be applied every time it gets restless. If the animal travels separately from its owner in a cage, start the treatment 15 days before the trip at a rate of 4 drops, six times per day, and on the day of the trip administer 4 drops every half hour until boarding time.

If the journey is short (no longer than an hour), prepare the animal by administering 4 drops every 15 minutes for an hour before leaving home, 4 drops just before getting into the car or other means of transport, and 4 drops at the end of the journey.

The Bach Flower formula recommended in these cases is the same as for visits to the vet and pre- and postoperative periods:

> Rescue Remedy (emergency) + Rock Rose (panic) + Star of Bethlehem (shock, trauma) + Sweet Chestnut (extreme anguish) + Olive (exhaustion) + Walnut (adaptation).

For animals that feel sick and vomit when they travel by car or other means of transport, add Scleranthus (instability) and Cherry Plum (lack of control) to the above formula instead of Rock Rose and Star of Bethlehem.

5.12 Pseudocyesis (psychological pregnancy)

Some female dogs enter a state called pseudocyesis or pseudopregnancy, where they have hormonal levels similar to those of a pregnant female, and these cause an anomalous behaviour in the dog. In order to give birth, the pseudopregnant female creates a kind of 'nest' with objects that she collects, and if there is another female near her that has given birth, she will try to nurse some of those puppies. Otherwise, she may adopt a shoe, small toy or other object, offering it the same loving and protective care that she would give to her own puppy.

This behaviour only occurs in female dogs and is a consequence of the type of evolution that the canine species has experienced. The dog is a descendant of the wolf and has inherited behaviours that have been passed on genetically. The wolf lives in herds composed of several females and one dominant male. The male is responsible for hunting and propagating the species by mating with the females of the group, while the females alternate hunting with taking care of their cubs.

Nature has provided the females of the canine species with the capacity to undergo pseudopregnancies, because when they go to find their own food, they delegate the nursing of their own young to other females of the same herd and this generates fictitious pregnancies in some of them.

A female dog with pseudopregnancy is hypersensitive, nervous and manifests changes in her appetite. It is usual for her to adopt a toy, pillow or shoe as a puppy. She may even imitate giving it food and warmth and become aggressive if an attempt is made to take it away.

We should let nature follow its course and treat the dog as if she were actually pregnant. It is important to accompany the process of pseudopregnancy with a Flower treatment that will cover different aspects of the maternal needs of a female dog. Among the most important to take into consideration are: possessiveness and excessive concern for the adopted object; near continuous attention seeking; and aggressiveness due to mistrust of those who approach her to take away her nonexistent puppy. Treatment of pseudopregnancy must also consider aspects of the learning process, that is, it should help the dog to avoid repeating the same process again and again. A female dog that manifests pseudopregnancy normally experiences it more than once, and this situation, besides having an impact on her emotional state, can lead to serious health problems due to the predominance of progestogens. Mastitis and diseases of the uterus, such as pyometra, a uterine infection that in acute cases can cause the death of the animal, are particularly dangerous. Therefore, pseudopregnancy in a female dog also requires vet visits and supervision.

Normally the pseudopregnancy occurs within two months after the female is in heat. As a preventive measure, the dog should be treated with the formula quoted below for approximately ten days after she is in heat, at a rate of 4 drops, four times per day.

The Bach Flowers recommended in the treatment of pseudocyesis are:

> Chestnut Bud (learning process) + Chicory (possessiveness of space, owner, objects, etc.) + Heather (demanding attention) + Red Chestnut (detachment) + Walnut (adaptation) + Rescue Remedy (if the dog is very restless) + Holly (if she shows signs of aggressiveness).

Depending on the case being treated, this formula should be administered at a rate of 4 drops, four to six or more times per day, in direct application whenever possible.

5.13 Socialization

5.13.1 Canine socialization

The socialization period comes approximately between the fourth and sixteenth week of an animal's life and is of vital importance, marking how it interacts with other animals and people for the rest of its life.

During this period the puppy shows an exceptional predisposition to learn and assimilate everything that happens around it. Between the sixth and eighth week of life the patterns that generate fear start, which the animal can perceive in a positive, negative or neutral way.

If during this period the puppy has little or no contact with people, it will react with fear or aggressiveness when it encounters a human in its adult stage. The same will happen if it hasn't spent time with other dogs as a puppy; as an adult it will react inappropriately when interacting with them.

Bach Flowers can help the animal that hasn't gone through the socialization process and complement the work of the professional who will teach it those socialization guidelines.

In order to treat these cases we need to consider the remedies that relate to learning issues. The actions of Chestnut Bud (learning process), Rock Water (resistance to change) and Walnut (adaptation) are essential tools for the canine trainer, behaviourist and Bach Flower Therapist. These remedies allow the animal to register new behavioural guidelines more quickly and assimilate the information received from the rest of the Flower formula's components more easily. An animal that is unable to socialize properly should also be administered Vervain, a remedy which will enhance its exploratory capabilities. These four remedies should be administered along with those that deal with the negative responses or anomalous behavioural patterns that the animal manifests towards another animal or human. Remember that to enhance learning capabilities we can also consider Cerato (trust and self-confidence), Clematis (facilitates attention) and Larch (disability).

The following Bach Flowers are recommended for treating canine lack of socialization:

> Chestnut Bud (learning process) + Rock Water (resistance to change) + Walnut (adaptation) + Vervain (exploratory capacity) + remedies that deal with the symptoms of lack of socialization.

Depending on the animal this formula should be administered at a rate of 4 drops, four to six times per day, for at least one month, in direct application if the animal shows no signs of aggressiveness.

5.13.2 Feline socialization

As in the case of dogs, it is also very important for cats to experience a proper socialization period in order to prevent possible behavioural problems as adults. During the first months of life, the cat develops and establishes its character and learns the behavioural patterns that will be necessary for it to establish peaceful relationships with other animals and humans.

Studies on feline behaviour show that a part of the psychomotor development of a cat begins before birth and has a strong genetic component, especially with regard to socialization with humans. Despite this, it is essential to educate it during the first six months of life. Educating an adult animal is possible but is more difficult and the success of the learning process would depend on its temperament and the teaching skills of the person in charge of educating it. Therefore, it is recommended that you seek the advice, assistance or services of a vet or feline behaviourist and treat the cat with a formula of Flower Remedies that work in synergy with the new guidelines it will receive.

To treat a cat's lack of socialization it is recommended that you use the formula that treats a dog's lack of socialization plus Beech, a remedy common to many cats, especially if the cat has to live with children or other animals.

A cat will often see a child as different from an adult. A child makes much more noise, treats the cat roughly and sometimes bothers it instead of playing. This obviously does not help the coexistence between the two of them.

The following Bach Flowers are recommended for treating feline lack of socialization:

> Beech (intolerance) + Chestnut Bud (learning process) + Rock Water (resistance to change) + Walnut (adaptation) + Vervain (exploratory capacity) + remedies that consider the cat's character + remedies that treat the negative symptoms of lack of socialization at an early age.

This formula should be administered at a rate of 4 drops, four to six or more times per day for at least one month, in direct application if the cat shows no signs of aggressiveness.

6

A SELECTION OF CASES TREATED

6.1 Aggressiveness

6.1.1 Fear-induced aggressiveness

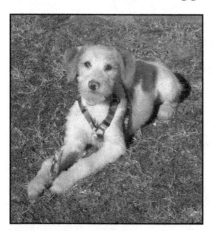

Name: Neula

Breed: Mixed

Sex: Female

Age / Imprinting:
3 months / lack of imprinting

Neula

REASON FOR CONSULTATION

Aggressiveness towards strangers and occasionally towards other animals. Neula's behaviourist diagnosed a behavioural problem compatible with a fear-induced agressiveness problem, normally directed towards strangers. Neula also manifested anxiety.

Neula was born in the Amics dels Animals de la Noguera shelter just days after her mother was found abandoned.

Shortly after being adopted she manifested aggressiveness toward strangers (see 'Fear-induced aggressiveness', p.106). The behavioural problem was more intense at home than outside; she would sometimes start barking at someone as if she were about to attack, and on other occasions she would pull back or avoid contact. This behaviour may be related to insufficient imprinting (see 'Canine and feline filial imprinting', p.124, and 'Canine socialization', p.132).

Neula was also afraid of being left alone and was constantly following her owners everywhere, showing signs of anxiety. For this reason, we also considered the remedies in the formula that treats separation anxiety (see 'Separation anxiety', p.111) in her treatment.

Remedies administered orally

(Refer to 'Preparation of a remedy for oral application', p.21.).

> Mimulus (fear) + Cherry Plum (lack of control) + Holly (mistrust) + Star of Bethlehem (trauma) + Walnut (adaptation) + Vervain (overexcitement) + White Chestnut (repetition).

The formula was administered at a rate of 4 drops, six times per day, in direct application.

Due to the fact that Neula manifested two different behavioural problems (aggressiveness and mild anxiety), in her first formula we combined remedies to manage fear-induced aggressiveness (the first three listed above) together with two remedies that managed her anxiety when left alone. Keep in mind that she was an animal born in a shelter and so the formula also dealt with traumatic after effects and her capacity to adapt.

After two months of treatment the level of aggressiveness was reduced and she was calmer, but signs of fear and anxiety were still present. At that time, Neula's owners decided to combine the Flower treatment with the advice of a canine trainer. Two new remedies were then added to her formula, Agrimony to strengthen the anxiolytic effect of the above-mentioned formula and Chestnut Bud to enhance her ability to learn and assimilate new guidelines. Holly was removed in order to avoid overloading the formula.

The new formula for Neula was as follows:

> Mimulus (fear) + Cherry Plum (lack of control) + Star of Bethlehem (trauma) + Walnut (adaptation) + Vervain (overexcitement) + White Chestnut (repetition) + Agrimony (anxiety) + Chestnut Bud (facilitates the learning process).

The formula was administered at a rate of 4 drops, six times per day, in direct application.

Three months after taking the new formula, and together with the change of guidelines from the canine trainer, Neula's level of anxiety was considerably improved and she presented a lower level of stress. We decided to remove Star of Bethlehem (trauma) and Walnut (adaptation) from the formula because we considered that these remedies had fulfilled their goal over the five months of treatment. Neula was now well adapted to her new family and home and manifested no traumatic after effects. However, Neula sometimes still showed signs of aggressiveness towards visitors. To help her in this aspect, we decided to add Rock Water (resistance to change) to her remedy combination.

The new formula administered to Neula is detailed below:

> Mimulus (fear) + Cherry Plum (lack of control) + Vervain (overexcitement) + White Chestnut (repetition) + Agrimony (anxiety) + Chestnut Bud (facilitates the learning process) + Rock Water (resistance to change).

It was administered at a rate of 4 drops, five times per day, in direct application.

This formula was maintained for three more months, a period in which Neula began to participate in discipline and rapport agility sessions with her trainer. Neula kept improving and responded positively to the discipline training. Her aggressive behaviour towards strangers and visitors also improved.

Observations

At present, Neula is continuing with the same Flower treatment and discipline training.

6.1.2 Canine redirected aggressiveness

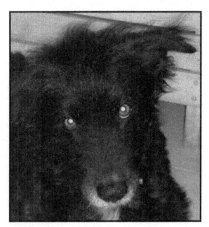

Name: Negret

Breed: Mixed

Sex: Male

Age / Imprinting:
4 years / lack of imprinting

Negret

Reason for consultation

Aggressiveness directed towards other male dogs and his owner during his daily walk in the park.

Negret and the dogs involved in the aggressiveness were kept on a lead by their owners. However, when Negret's owner tried to hold him back, he directed his aggressiveness towards her (see 'Territorial, possessive and redirected aggressiveness', p.108).

Negret also showed excitement and nervousness every time his owner returned home, demanding her continuous attention.

Remedies administered orally

(Refer to 'Preparation of a remedy for oral application', p.21.).

> Holly (rage) + Beech (intolerance) + Cherry Plum (lack of control, hysteria) + Vine (domination) + Chicory (possessiveness of space, owners, objects, etc.) + Heather (demanding attention) + Rescue Remedy (emergency).

The formula was administered at a rate of 4 drops, five times per day, in direct application.

Negret's formula combines remedies to treat redirected aggressiveness. The first five are remedies that deal with the type of relationship he has established with his owner. He was also administered Rescue Remedy to calm him down.

After two and a half months Negret's behaviour had improved considerably. When faced with another male dog he was on the alert but not aggressive. He felt stressed when near dogs he had previously fought with but did not turn on his owner to bite her. Now, when the owner tells him off he obeys quickly, and he is generally calmer, especially when she returns home. He does not scratch the doors, and neither barks nor jumps hysterically. Despite his positive initial response, Negret continued treatment with the same formula for two more months.

6.1.3 Feline fear-induced aggressiveness

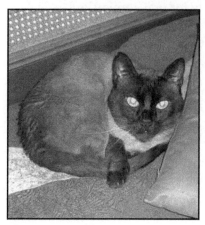

Name: Miki

Breed: Siamese

Sex: Male

Age / Imprinting:
8 years / lack of imprinting.
Was taken from the litter
when he was barely one
month old.

Miki

REASON FOR CONSULTATION

*Fear-induced aggressiveness and tendency to withdraw from familiar
people or strangers.*

Miki was a very unfriendly and fearful animal, and was terrified
by any small noise.

Except for his owner, no one could approach to pet him. He
hissed and scratched in order to defend himself (see 'Fear-induced
aggressiveness', p.106). Together with fear-induced aggressiveness
he had a significant tendency to withdraw to his isolation fields.
The isolation fields (as referred to in the oral application of Water
Violet, p.93) are the areas to which an animal withdraws to avoid
contact with people and/or other animals. Most cats choose three
areas of isolation. Miki's isolation zones were radiators, inside a
cupboard and under the covers of his owner's bed. He normally
slept in these places and also used them as a refuge when he was in
a situation that he interpreted as dangerous (e.g. someone visiting
the house, the owner's relative's dogs coming, etc.). Miki always
chose places that were high up in order to isolate himself. He
rarely hid under the bed.

Remedies administered orally
(Refer to 'Preparation of a remedy for oral application', p.21.)

> Mimulus (fear) + Rock Rose (panic) + Star of Bethlehem (trauma, shock) + Holly (jealousy) + Beech (intolerance, rejection) + Cherry Plum (lack of control, hysteria) + Water Violet (significant withdrawal to isolation field).

The treatment was given in indirect application.

Due to Miki's fearful nature and his aggressive warning signals (meowing, hissing and trying to scratch) when someone, even his owner, went to pick him up, we decided not to give the 4 drops of each dose directly into his mouth, but through indirect application (see 'Indirect application', p.29).

Miki had improved significantly 15 days after beginning the treatment. When a relative or an acquaintance visited the owner, Miki still isolated himself but chose his isolation area in the same room as the visitors. If they were in the living room, he took refuge on the radiator or on top of the sofa instead of running away to the bedroom where, before the Flower treatment, he used to isolate himself from any person other than his owner.

After approximately one month he did not manifest fear at the arrival of the owner's relative's dogs. He observed the dogs from the top of the sofa, but remained relaxed. In the past, when confronted with the same dogs he would quickly hide or jump somewhere higher than ground level (e.g. the radiator or the sofa's head-rest). With the help of Flower Therapy, Miki has increased his level of socialization with people and other animals, and has decreased the time spent in areas that constitute his isolation field.

The treatment was interrupted after two months of using the same Flower formula. Twelve days later he returned to his old patterns of isolation and fear-induced aggressiveness. This indicates that this problem requires a longer course of treatment before the remedies are completely effective, so we recommend that treatment should last at least six months in cases where the behavioural problem has existed since the animal was very young.

Currently Miki has been under continuous treatment for seven months and is expected to continue his treatment for at least five more months.

6.1.4 Feline redirected aggressiveness

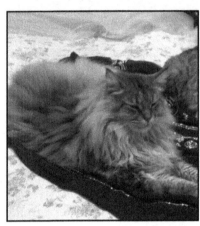

Name: Linus

Breed: Maine Coon

Sex: Male

Age / Imprinting:
8 years / yes

Linus

REASON FOR CONSULTATION

Redirected aggressiveness induced by change.

Linus showed signs of aggressiveness since his owner separated from her partner, even when he sometimes returned to visit them. After two years, his aggressive behaviour worsened when his owner adopted another cat and started a new relationship. Linus didn't accept his owner's new boyfriend and prevented him from entering the house. Linus remained at the door, blocking the way while hissing at him. One day he attacked his owner, causing her medium-level injuries (see 'Territorial, possessive and redirected aggressiveness', p.108).

Remedies administered orally

(Refer to 'Preparation of a remedy for oral application', p. 21.)

> Holly (jealousy, hypersensitivity) + Beech (intolerance, rejection) + Cherry Plum (lack of control, hysteria) + Vine (domination) + Willow (resentment) + Walnut (adaptation).

The recommended dose is 4 drops, four times per day, in direct application.

This formula was given to Linus for two months. At the end of this period an improvement in his aggressive behaviour was noted. There were no new attacks towards the owner. However, he still prevented the owner's partner from entering the house on approximately half of his visits.

Due to the owner's work timetable, she could only administer the remedies twice a day instead of four times as recommended. This may be one of the factors why the problem was not solved. It was decided that the frequency of the dosage would be increased to four times per day, even though this involved giving two doses in a row in the morning (before the owner left the house) and two doses in a row at night (when she returned from work). We also decided to add Chicory (possessiveness) to the above-mentioned formula to manage Linus's excessive possessiveness towards his owner.

During the third month Linus was administered the following formula:

> Holly (jealousy, hypersensitivity) + Beech (intolerance, rejection) + Cherry Plum (lack of control, hysteria) + Vine (domination) + Willow (resentment) + Walnut (adaptation) + Chicory (possessiveness).

A slight improvement was achieved compared with the first formula, but it was still not sufficient. Linus did not attack his owner any more but still continued to hold off her partner.

We suggested that the owner use the same formula for one more month, but this time combining direct application (see 'Direct application', p.27) at a rate of 4 drops, four times a day, with indirect application (see 'Indirect application', p.29). After this time we observed slight changes, but never beyond the 60 per cent improvement threshold.

OBSERVATIONS

After four months of treatment without completely solving Linus's aggressive attitude, the owner decided to stop the treatment.

6.1.5 Canine possessive aggressiveness

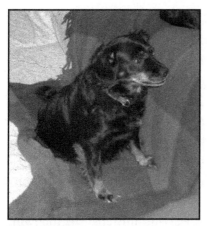

Nora

Name: Nora

Breed: Mixed

Sex: Female

Age / Imprinting:
10 years / unknown

REASON FOR CONSULTATION

Aggressiveness directed at people trying to approach her owner.

Nora had never been a very sociable dog with other animals (except for a brother from the same litter) or with people who visited her owners. She had never attacked anyone, but she would usually growl in front of a stranger or acquaintance, and would not let anyone come close. As time went by, she began to show possessiveness towards her owner by increasingly preventing neighbours from approaching her. One day she almost bit a neighbour (see 'Territorial, possessive and redirected aggressiveness', p.108).

Remedies administered orally

(Refer to 'Preparation of a remedy for oral application', p.21.)

> Holly (jealousy) + Beech (intolerance, rejection) + Vine (domination) + Chicory (possessiveness).

The formula was administered at a rate of 4 drops, four times per day, in direct application.

A few days after Nora started to take the remedies she manifested eczema on her skin and small areas of alopecia. Crab Apple (cleansing) was added to the formula and development was monitored.

Within a week her possessive behaviour and consequent aggressiveness towards the owner had improved considerably. Only occasionally did she show some signs of aggressiveness, usually warning people not to approach her.

Despite this rapid improvement the formula was administered for two more months, achieving full remission of her behavioural problem.

Observations

Nora died of a cirrhotic liver problem two years later.

6.1.6 Canine secondary aggressiveness

Name: Brauli

Breed: Mixed

Sex: Male

Age / Imprinting: 2 years / unknown

REASON FOR CONSULTATION

Brauli manifests secondary aggressiveness when having his skin wounds treated.

Brauli was found in a deplorable condition in an abandoned factory. He had problems with the vision in both his eyes, areas of alopecia on his body and infected wounds, and he was very thin and exhausted. When rescued, he showed no signs of aggressiveness, but later manifested secondary aggressiveness each time he underwent daily care and treatment of his wounds (see 'Secondary aggressiveness', p.109).

REMEDIES ADMINISTERED ORALLY

(Refer to 'Preparation of a remedy for oral application', p.21.)

> Rescue Remedy (emergency) + Cherry Plum (lack of control, hysteria) + Elm (pain sensitive to touch) + Star of Bethlehem (shock) + Mimulus (fear) + Olive (exhaustion, revitalizing).

The first day the formula was administered to Brauli in indirect application, as he showed signs of aggressiveness when approached. From the second day onwards both types of application were combined (with direct application at a rate of 4 drops, two times per day). As he became more trusting towards his owner, the number of doses could be increased, reaching a maximum of six times per day.

This formula combined remedies that treat secondary aggressiveness (the first four listed above) with remedies that manage the fear and devitalization that Brauli manifested from the first day of rescue.

After three days using this formula Brauli improved greatly and he stopped holding off the owner whenever he tried to treat his wounds. Two months later he recovered sight in both eyes and had only a few areas of alopecia.

OBSERVATIONS

Simultaneously with the oral treatment, the areas with alopecia and infected wounds were treated by applying a cream with the remedies listed below:

> Rescue Remedy (emergency) + Crab Apple (cleanse) + Star of Bethlehem (cicatrizant, shock expressed through alopecia) + Hornbeam (local energy) + Olive (revitalizer).

Local treatment, applied three times daily, began on the fourth day after starting oral treatment.

6.2 Anxiety

6.2.1 Separation anxiety

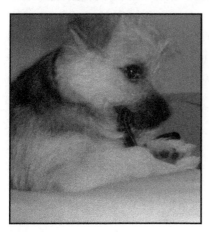

Name: Joss

Breed: Mixed

Sex: Male

Age / Imprinting:
1 and a half years / unknown

Joss

REASON FOR CONSULTATION

Arrhythmia.

Joss is a hyperactive dog that suffered separation anxiety (see 'Separation anxiety', p.111) which subsequently manifested as arrhythmia. The vet prescribed Clomicalm (an anxiolytic) and recommended that a series of behavioural guidelines be put into practice every time the owners went to work or returned home, two situations that involved a lot of excitement for Joss.

However, no improvement was observed with this treatment. Joss constantly followed the owners everywhere. When they went to work he cried, barked and scratched the door. When they returned in the afternoon he would go crazy and out of control. He had recently experienced a house move.

In order to help Joss feel less lonely, his owners adopted a female puppy and decided to try Bach Flowers.

Remedies administered orally
(Refer to 'Preparation of a remedy for oral application', p.21.)

> Rescue Remedy (emergency) + Sweet chestnut (extreme anguish) + Walnut (adaptation) + Heather (demanding attention) + Vervain (overexcitement) + Cherry Plum (lack of control, hysteria).

The formula was administered at a rate of 4 drops, four times per day, in direct application.

A day after starting the remedies Joss was even more anxious. We decided to reduce the number of doses from four to two times per day for one week and then continue with the initial frequency.

Fifteen days later Joss's progress was quite positive. When his owners made a certain movement indicating they were preparing to leave home, Joss stayed on the alert but he did not get stressed. On the owners' return home, Joss's level of excitement decreased but still remained at a medium/low level.

The same formula was continued for approximately two months after treatment started, until Joss manifested a new behavioural problem: jealousy towards the female puppy. It seemed like Joss had gone back to being a puppy. He behaved in the same way as the puppy and showed signs of aggressiveness when reprimanded. Holly (jealousy) was added to the new formula, as follows:

> Rescue Remedy (emergency) + Sweet Chestnut (extreme anguish) + Walnut (adaptation) + Heather (demanding attention) + Vervain (overexcitement) + Cherry Plum (lack of control, hysteria) + Holly (jealousy).

The new formula was administered at a rate of 4 drops, five times per day, in direct application.

After three months of treatment the owners reported that Joss was more sensitive, constantly wanting to be near them when they were at home. He did not want to sleep on his blanket at night and repeatedly jumped on their bed, not having done this so insistently before. A new formula was prepared for Joss that substituted Chicory (possessiveness) for Walnut, as follows:

> Rescue Remedy (emergency) + Sweet Chestnut (extreme anguish) + Heather (demanding attention) + Vervain (overexcitement) + Cherry Plum (lack of control, hysteria) + Holly (jealousy) + Chicory (possessiveness).

It was administered at a rate of 4 drops, five times per day, in direct application.

After four months of treatment Joss's separation anxiety and demand for attention had remitted completely.

6.2.2 Separation anxiety

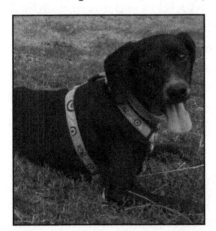

Name: Nuki

Breed: Cocker-Labrador cross

Sex: Female

Age / Imprinting:
2 years / unknown

Nuki

REASON FOR CONSULTATION

Separation anxiety and destructive behaviour after moving with her owner to another apartment.

Nuki lived with her owner at her owner's parents' house. When she was about one year old, her owner changed job and they both went to live in a different city. Her owner now had less free time to spend with her and take her for walks. From then, she began manifesting symptoms of anxiety when left alone at home, urinating and defecating on the floor and destroying shoes, toys and other objects, and when her owner returned, she manifested excessive overexcitement (see 'Separation anxiety', p.111).

Remedies administered orally
(Refer to 'Preparation of a remedy for oral application', p.21.)

> Chicory (possessiveness) + Heather (demanding attention) + Agrimony (anxiety) + Impatiens (acceleration) + Vervain (overexcitement) + Mimulus (fear) + Walnut (adaptation) + Sweet Chestnut (extreme anguish).

The formula was administered at a rate of 4 drops, a minimum of four times per day, in direct application. The daily frequency of Nuki's treatment was subject to her owner's working hours, which varied every day.

After one month of treatment with this formula, Nuki's anxiety level had dropped considerably. When left alone she did not break or destroy anything and only defecated and urinated in the house on rare occasions. The formula was repeated for one more month, administering it four times per day, and Nuki's anxiety syndrome ceased completely. Nevertheless, we decided to prolong the treatment for one more month but at a low frequency of a minimum of two times per day.

Although eight months have elapsed since Nuki stopped her treatment with Flower Remedies, she has not since shown any signs of anxiety when left alone at home.

6.3 Jealousy
6.3.1 Early maternal rejection of puppies

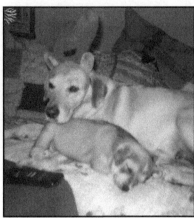

Name: Wilma

Breed: Labrador

Sex: Female

Age / Imprinting:
7 years / lack of imprinting

Wilma

Reason for consultation

Attitude of rejection towards her puppies and aggressiveness towards one in particular.

Wilma would growl at her puppies when they approached her in order to feed. She even bit off a piece of one of the puppies' ears. Wilma had always been possessive with her owner, and when the owner paid attention to the puppies Wilma became upset, manifesting her jealousy and anger.

Wilma lived with her owner from when she was two months old and as a puppy she was very shy and fearful.

Remedies administered orally

(Refer to 'Preparation of a remedy for oral application', p.21.)

> Chicory (possessiveness) + Beech (intolerance, rejection) + Heather (demanding attention) + Holly (jealousy) + Vine (territoriality) + Walnut (adaptation) + Chestnut Bud (facilitates the learning process).

The formula was administered at a rate of 4 drops, five times per day, in direct application.

After a week's treatment Wilma's behaviour had improved. She started to let her puppies approach her to nurse and gradually started to carry out the normal functions of a female who has just given birth. She also accepted the attention that the puppies received from her owner and visitors better. Nevertheless, as a precaution, treatment was extended for another month.

Two years after the treatment ended we got in touch with Wilma's owner who informed us that Wilma had established an excellent relationship with Kalcio, the female puppy (crossed with a husky) that was the subject of Wilma's attacks when she was a small puppy.

OBSERVATIONS

After approximately a month of nursing her pups, Wilma presented with mastitis which was treated with a local remedy (see Case 7.8, p.206).

6.3.2 Feline jealousy-induced aggressiveness

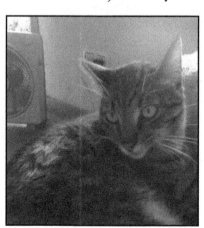

Name: Eko

Breed: Domestic shorthaired

Sex: Male

Age / Imprinting:
1 year / lack of imprinting

Eko

REASON FOR CONSULTATION

Aggressiveness induced by jealousy towards the arrival of a new animal in the family.

Eko is a cat that was separated from the litter when he was two months old and easily adapted to his new home. He had a fearful character, yet at the same time he was playful and possessive with his owners. When the family had someone visit for too long, Eko would nip the visitor. He was also unfriendly and hissed at his owners' children and grandchildren, even though they visited frequently. Furthermore, he didn't like anybody sitting next to his owner. However, the serious behavioural problem occurred when a new cat temporarily came into the family. When Eko saw the new arrival he hissed and scratched it. Eko even started being aggressive with the family (see 'Feline social aggression', p.110, and 'Territorial, possessive and redirected aggressiveness', p.108).

Although the second cat was returned, Eko continued to behave aggressively with his family for one month, even with his owner, with whom he had had a very good relationship before the arrival of the 'intruder'. He even hissed and bit occasionally.

We decided to start a Flower treatment to address simultaneously both types of aggressiveness together with his possessive and fearful character, even though this involved using eight remedies in the formula. The first two remedies addressed his typology (character type). The following three dealt with the way Eko experienced the arrival of the new family member and also how he expressed his dissatisfaction, even though the second cat no longer lived with them. The last three remedies addressed Eko's resistance to change, and also his lack of adaptation and assimilation towards a new cat and towards his owners' relatives and visitors.

Remedies administered orally

(Refer to 'Preparation of a remedy for oral application', p.21.)

> Chicory (possessiveness) + Mimulus (fear) + Beech (intolerance, rejection) + Holly (jealousy) + Willow (resentment) + Chestnut Bud (facilitates the learning process) + Rock Water (resistance to change) + Walnut (adaptation).

On days when Eko's family did not expect visitors the formula was applied at a rate of 4 drops, five times per day. Four hours before the arrival of the owners' relatives or acquaintances the formula was applied at a rate of 4 drops every half hour. Both options were applied in direct application.

After ten days of treatment Eko's level of aggressiveness towards the family members decreased considerably; he started to tolerate the children and grandchildren when they visited. The hissing stopped completely, and after one month Eko showed no signs of any type of aggressiveness, sometimes even sitting on his owners' son's lap.

We continued the same formula for one more month and then we decided the treatment was finished.

6.4 Feline idiopathic cystitis

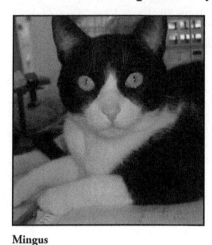

Name: Mingus

Breed: Domestic shorthaired

Sex: Male

Age / Imprinting:
6 years / yes

Mingus

Reason for consultation

Recurrent infections of the urinary tract after visits to the vet.

Mingus was a quiet and affectionate cat with a rather fearful nature. He would quickly hide when he heard any noise.

After castration, Mingus would get very nervous on each visit to the vet, trembling throughout, and three days later the stress would manifest as a urine infection (see 'Stress-related urine infections', p.126).

The vet checked his kidneys for any serious pathology but the urine analysis showed only the presence of grit in the kidney.

Remedies administered by indirect application

(Refer to 'Preparation of a remedy for oral application', p.21, and 'Indirect application', p.29).

> Star of Bethlehem (shock, trauma) + Rock Rose (panic) + Mimulus (fear) + Crab Apple (cleanse) + Olive (exhaustion due to stress) + Walnut (adaptation to change).

As a preventive treatment we decided to use this formula approximately ten days before the visit to the vet in indirect application. During Mingus's next visit to the vet he was calmer than on other occasions and he did not contract a new urine infection afterwards. He did, however, develop an infection on his tail. We decided to give him the same formula orally at a rate of 4 drops, four times per day. Within days this infection had disappeared.

Observations

It was recommended that a preventive treatment with this formula be given to Mingus approximately ten days before each annual vaccination or any routine visit to the vet.

Any stressful situation (see 'Stress', p.121) activates the animal's sympathetic nervous system, and hence its adrenal glands, causing immediate secretion of cortisol. If this situation lasts for a long period of time, on a continuous basis, it may produce a dysfunction of these glands that affects the animal's mood and immune system.

6.5 Coprophagia

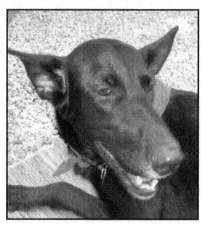

Name: Nica

Breed: Belgian Shepherd cross

Sex: Female

Age / Imprinting:
2 years / unknown

Nica

REASON FOR CONSULTATION

Separation anxiety and coprophagia.

After a visit to the vet, Nica was diagnosed with separation anxiety and coprophagia. She manifested a high level of anxiety, eating everything she found in the street including excrement (see 'Coprophagia', p.115). She also barked at every dog that passed by, and if approached she would hold them off by growling. This behavioural problem seemed to be more a case of attention-seeking rather than aggressiveness. Nica also expressed fear of being left alone at home, an inherent behaviour of separation anxiety (see 'Separation anxiety', p.111).

REMEDIES ADMINISTERED ORALLY

(Refer to 'Preparation of a remedy for oral application', p.21.)

> Chicory (possessiveness) + Heather (demanding attention) + Agrimony (anxiety) + Impatiens (acceleration) + Mimulus (fear) + Beech (intolerance, rejection of other animals) + Chestnut Bud (learning process).

The formula was administered at a rate of 4 drops, four times per day, in direct application.

Three days after starting the treatment, Nica's need to be the centre of attention had increased; she was not only barking at dogs when walking in the street, but was also barking at them from the balcony. We decided to continue with the same treatment and at the same frequency. Seven days later this behaviour improved greatly.

The formula was maintained for two more months and after this time Nica's separation anxiety had improved significantly, showing lower levels of stress. The problem of coprophagia had also improved.

To further improve the coprophagia issue, which was a consequence of her anxiety levels, we decided to add Rescue Remedy to the formula. As her attitude towards other dogs improved, Beech was removed.

Nica's new formula was as follows:

> Chicory (possessiveness) + Heather (demanding attention) + Agrimony (anxiety) + Impatiens (acceleration) + Mimulus (fear) + Chestnut Bud (learning process) + Rescue Remedy.

It was administered at a rate of 4 drops, four times per day in direct application.

After two months of treatment with this formula, Nica's anxiety level had dropped and her problem of coprophagia had improved.

Observations

Nica's owner decided to give up the therapy after four months of treatment, due to issues at work.

6.6 Defecation and urination in inappropriate places

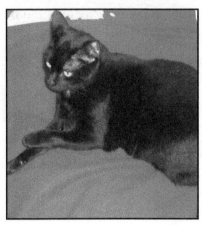

Name: Taika

Breed: Domestic shorthaired

Sex: Female

Age / Imprinting:
8 years / unknown

Taika

REASON FOR CONSULTATION

Defecation and urination in inappropriate places.

Taika was a very affectionate cat and demanded constant attention from her owner. She had an elimination disorder (see 'Defecation and urination in inappropriate places', p.118) that worsened when her owner had visitors. The problem reached its most acute phase when Taika's owner's parents came to stay for a week. During that period of time, Taika began to express dissatisfaction towards her owner by defecating around the house, on one occasion defecating on the visitors' bed. Finally, one day Taika sat on her owner's lap as she usually did when she sat on the sofa, but this time she urinated on her skirt.

Remedies administered orally

(Refer to 'Preparation of a remedy for oral application', p.21.)

> Chicory (possessiveness) + Heather (demanding attention) + Holly (jealousy) + Vine (domination) + Beech (intolerance and rejection).

The formula was administered at a rate of 4 drops, four times per day, in direct application.

After one month of treatment Taika's elimination disorder and behaviour had improved very little. However, after adding Willow to her formula, the defecation and urination in inappropriate places stopped completely.

Observations

Taika died of mammary cancer one year later.

6.7 Kidney failure

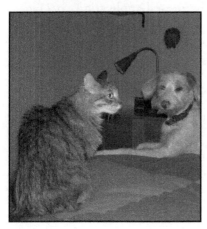

Name: Max

Breed: Domestic cross

Sex: Male

Age / Imprinting:
6 years / unknown

Max

REASON FOR CONSULTATION

Kidney failure and fear due to the arrival of a new animal in the home.

Max was adopted when he was about five months old. A lady saw him fall out of the window of a building and picked him up; he had probably slipped off the windowsill. She took him to the vet where he was found a new home.

Despite the fact that Max surprisingly only broke a tooth, he also experienced a significant emotional shock in the fall. From the beginning Max was a very fearful and unfriendly animal. Of course, it is impossible to know if these characteristics result from the emotional impact suffered by the fall, or if they were part of his intrinsic nature. When Max was approximately four years old, he was diagnosed with kidney failure on a routine visit to the vet, a condition requiring medication and a special diet.

A year later, Max's owners adopted a two-month-old female dog (Neula; see Case 6.1.1, p.137) from an animal shelter. This arrival of a new animal into the house significantly worsened Max's fearful nature. He reacted by hiding away in a room, not wanting to go out, and spending most of the day under the bed.

Remedies administered orally

(Refer to 'Preparation of a remedy for oral application', p.21.)

> Mimulus (fear) + Rock Rose (panic) + Star of Bethlehem (shock) + Beech (intolerance and rejection) + Walnut (adaptation) + Olive (exhaustion, devitalization) + Gorse (submission).

The formula was administered at a rate of 4 drops, four times per day, in direct application.

Max's formula treated his fearful nature and the traumatic panic he experienced with his new housemate, Neula. The formula also included Olive and Gorse to energetically strengthen the kidney area. According to Traditional Chinese Medicine, experiencing situations of fear and panic 'exhausts' the kidney.

One month later Max was still in his owner's room. However, Max now defended his space by challenging Neula. After three months of treatment his fearful attitude of avoiding the puppy had improved considerably. It must be emphasized that the puppy's insistent playful attitude considerably helped Max to adapt to the new situation. Despite this improvement we decided to extend the treatment in order to prevent Max becoming more stressed by the puppy's constant urge to play. Neula manifested separation anxiety, and when left alone she would seek the company of Max.

After just over a year of pharmacological and Flower treatment, and following the relevent tests, the vet informed Max's owner that he no longer had kidney failure.

In most cases where a cat suffers from kidney failure, the condition becomes chronic. It rarely remits, even when treated with appropriate medication. Kidney failure occurs when the kidneys cannot remove waste products from the blood. These accumulate and produce clinical symptoms associated with kidney diseases, such as poor appetite, weight loss, increased thirst and vomiting. The kidneys cannot concentrate the urine or absorb enough water to be returned to the bloodstream. This leads to dehydration and the production of diluted urine, which tends to increase the frequency of urination during the day and produce nighttime urination.

6.8 Leishmaniasis

How Bach Flowers can help during the process of this disease

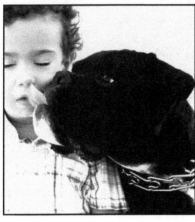

Lola

Name: Lola

Breed: Boxer

Sex: Female

Age / Imprinting:
15 months / unknown

REASON FOR CONSULTATION

Leishmaniasis.

Leishmaniasis is a disease caused by a parasite (phlebotomus) transmitted by a mosquito bite. The parasite invades different organs in the dog causing lesions of varying degrees and can be fatal.

The disease has a very diverse clinical symptomatology, but we highlight the following: skin lesions (alopecia, scabbing, ulcers), lesions in the joints, weight loss, muscle atrophy, haemorrhages, increase in the size of liver and spleen, limping and, when the disease is in an advanced state, signs of kidney failure. The ulcers are mainly located on different parts of the head (snout, ears, area around the eyes, etc.).

Remedies administered orally

(Refer to 'Preparation of a remedy for oral application', p.21.)

> Crab Apple (cleanse) + Centaury (weakness and domination
> by the parasite) + Olive (exhaustion, devitalization) + Gorse
> (for its positive effect on the immune system) + Scleranthus
> (cyclicity of the disease) + Rescue Remedy (emergency).

The formula was administered at a rate of 4 drops, five times per day for eight months, in direct application.

Lola was treated simultaneously with medication and Flower Remedies. After eight months, her antibody count had decreased from 640 to 160.

6.9 Feline chronic megacolon and megaoesophagus

Name: Lolita

Breed: Siamese

Sex: Female

Age / Imprinting: 7 years / unknown

REASON FOR CONSULTATION

Chronic megacolon. Difficulty defecating normally.

Lolita is a cat that was found abandoned at a train station; she was very frightened and presented many physical problems.

When an animal has a megacolon, its excrement accumulates as bags inside the colon, making elimination difficult. In Lolita's case the problem worsened because she also had megaoesophagus. The alimentary bolus (the mass of food that after mastication enters the oesophagus at one swallow) built up in the oesophagus, distending and increasing its size and not completing the passage into the stomach. Lolita frequently vomited due to difficulty digesting food.

Despite receiving pharmacological treatment (antibiotics, anti-inflammatory and anti-vomiting drugs), Lolita's problem did not improve. She was increasingly malnourished and in a low emotional state.

Lolita's Flower treatment addressed three important aspects. First, we included remedies that physically and energetically revitalized Lolita and remedies that enabled her not to surrender. This was helpful in improving her low physical and emotional state, which was essential for Lolita to be able to overcome her problem. Second, we included remedies that managed her resistance to keeping food inside the oesophagus (if she vomited she did not nourish herself and got weaker and weaker), and remedies that helped excretion (thereby preventing recurrent intestinal infections). Third, the formula addressed her fear and traumatic panic that came mainly as a result of having been abandoned.

REMEDIES ADMINISTERED ORALLY

(Refer to 'Preparation of a remedy for oral application', p.21.)

> Olive (exhaustion, devitalization) + Gorse (submission, boost to the immune system) + Willow (retention) + Beech (intolerance, rejection) + Crab Apple (obstruction and cleanse) + Rock Rose (panic) + Star of Bethlehem (shock, trauma) + Mimulus (fear).

The formula was administered at a rate of 4 drops, four times per day, in direct application.

After one month Lolita's problems had improved. She vomited less frequently and gained weight. We decided to remove Willow (retention) and add Chicory (congestion, retention) to help with Lolita's difficulty with excretion and possessive character. Lolita's formula was therefore as follows:

> Olive (devitalization) + Gorse (submission, boost to the immune system) + Beech (intolerance, rejection) + Crab Apple (obstruction and cleanse) + Rock Rose (panic) + Star of Bethlehem (shock, trauma) + Mimulus (fear) + Chicory (congestion, retention).

It was administered at a rate of 4 drops, four times per day, in direct application.

After the second month of treatment, Lolita's physical problems and fearful behaviour continued to improve. We decided to withdraw Mimulus and Beech from the formula and add Chestnut Bud (assimilation) in order to maintain the results we had obtained.

Below is the formula that Lolita is currently taking:

Olive (revitalizer) + Gorse (submission, boost to the immune system) + Crab Apple (obstruction and cleanse) + Rock Rose (panic) + Star of Bethlehem (shock, trauma) + Chicory (congestion, retention) + Chestnut Bud (assimilation).

It is administered at a rate of 4 drops, four times per day, in direct application.

Lolita is currently being treated with this Flower formula and is progressing favourably.

6.10 Fear and panic

6.10.1 Noise-induced fear and panic (fireworks)

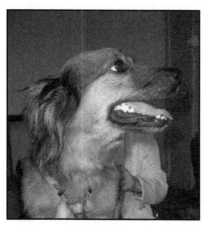

Name: Luna

Breed: Mixed

Sex: Female

Age / Imprinting:
6 years / unknown

Luna

Reason for consultation

After effects of post-traumatic panic.

Luna had hidden under the bed and refused to come out of her owner's room since Barcelona Football Club won both the league and European Cup on the same day, when she was subjected to very loud noises (klaxons, firecrackers, drums and people shouting). Luna apparently disliked so much 'happiness'. From that moment on she became more fearful.

Remedies administered orally

(Refer to 'Preparation of a remedy for oral application', p.21.)

> Mimulus (fear) + Rock Rose (panic) + Star of Bethlehem (shock, trauma) + Rescue Remedy (emergency).

The formula was administered at a rate of 4 drops, four to five times per day, in direct application.

During the first month of treatment Luna's behaviour improved. She didn't hide under the bed any more but was still on the alert when she heard normal sounds of domestic life. Her stress level decreased. We asked her owner to evaluate Luna's improvement on a scale of 0 to 10 and she gave a 7. To reduce her stress level further, we decided to add Sweet Chestnut (extreme anguish) to the new formula. Below is the new formula that was prepared:

Mimulus (fear) + Rock Rose (panic) + Star of Bethlehem (shock) + Rescue Remedy (emergency) + Sweet Chestnut (extreme anguish).

It was administered at a rate of 4 drops, four times per day, in direct application.

This formula was administered for another month and the owner reported that Luna's improvement level had increased from a 7 to an 8.

We decided to extend the treatment for one more month with the same formula plus the Walnut (adaptation) at a rate of 4 drops, four times per day. Luna's owner then went on holiday for a few weeks leaving Luna with a relative, at which time the treatment ended.

It is highly recommended, and I would say essential, that animals that have suffered this type of trauma receive a preventive treatment whenever there is a celebration accompanied by fireworks in the neighbourhood or city. It is sufficient to begin treatment one week before the event, at a rate of 4 drops, four to six times per day. On the day before and the day of the celebration administer the formula very frequently – every five minutes if the animal requires it and the owner's time availability allows. Finally, continue the treatment for two to three days after the end of the stress-inducing event (see Section 5.8, p.121).

6.10.2 Noise-induced fear and panic (house renovation)

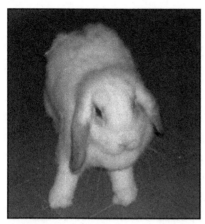

Name: Piccola

Breed: Belier (Rabbit)

Sex: Female

Age / Imprinting:
8 months / yes

Piccola

REASON FOR CONSULTATION

After effects of post-traumatic panic.

Piccola is a rabbit that showed frightened and aggressive behaviour following very loud house renovation work in the adjoining house. From then on, Piccola reacted aggressively every time people attempted to hold or feed her.

REMEDIES ADMINISTERED ORALLY

(Refer to 'Preparation of a remedy for oral application', p.21.)

> Mimulus (fear) + Rock Rose (panic) + Star of Bethlehem (trauma, shock) + Cherry Plum (lack of control, hysteria).

The formula was administered at a rate of 4 drops, two times per day, in direct application in combination with indirect application.

Although direct application is generally more effective than indirect application, we decided to combine them both because Piccola behaved aggressively when people tried to hold her. Holding Piccola four times per day in order to apply treatment meant putting the animal under too much stress.

Three weeks after starting the treatment Piccola had improved considerably. She was not as scared, but she still showed signs of mistrust and aggressiveness.

It came as a surprise when, after one month of taking the Flowers, she manifested an aggressive outburst, lightly biting her owner while she was feeding her. As this was a one-off event we did not consider changing the formula, but decided to administer it only through indirect application for a week to prevent further aggressive episodes. During this period of time Piccola did not show any sign of aggressiveness. On the contrary, she accepted a minimum of petting and stroking. From then on, we decided to administer the remedies only in direct application at a rate of 4 drops, four times per day until completing a treatment period of three months.

Piccola no longer shows any signs of aggressiveness. She likes being petted and accepts being held.

6.10.3 Fear and panic induced by mistreatment and abandonment

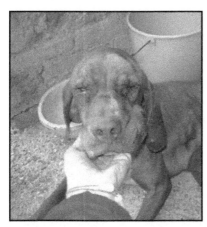

Misia

Name: Misia

Breed: Mixed (hunting dog)

Sex: Female

Age / Imprinting:
2 years / unknown

Reason for consultation

After effects of post-traumatic panic.

Misia was found in deplorable conditions: she was very malnourished, the skin on her abdomen was completely irritated and had an open wound, and the area around her eyes was red and swollen. She also presented infectious conjunctivitis and was in heat. The veterinarian certified that she had been poisoned and was suffering from a fairly high degree of malnutrition. After being hospitalized for several days in a veterinary clinic she was admitted to the Amics dels Animals de la Noguera animal shelter.

Besides presenting a general state of panic, her face expressed despair, exhaustion and great sadness.

Remedies administered orally

(Refer to 'Preparation of a remedy for oral application', p.21.)

Mimulus (fear) + Rock Rose (panic) + Star of Bethlehem (trauma) + Crab Apple (cleanse) + Gorse (submission) + Mustard (sadness, depression) + Olive (exhaustion).

The formula was administered for three weeks at a rate of 4 drops, four times per day, in direct application combined with indirect application.

After six days of treatment Misia had improved greatly. She had put on weight and her expression was no longer one of despair or sadness. She was also not so afraid when approached by volunteers from the shelter.

Misia was very lucky: about three weeks after arriving at the shelter she was adopted by a family. Treatment was continued for two more weeks and the owners reported that Misia did not have any adaptation problems.

6.10.4 Fear and panic due to mistreatment

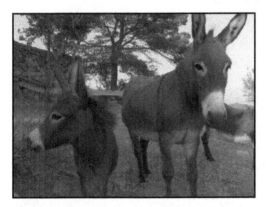

Name: Bony and Ruc

Breed: Donkeys

Sex: Males

Age / Imprinting: 3 years / unknown

Bony and Ruc

Reason for consultation

Fear and panic due to mistreatment.

Bony and Ruc were two donkeys that were raised in Mallorca. Their current owner had bought them at a cattle market. Bony's appearance was deplorable. He had been beaten and suffered damage to one eye. Both donkeys were panic-stricken and nobody could approach them.

Remedies administered orally

(Refer to 'Preparation of a remedy for oral application', p.21.)

> Rock Rose (panic) + Mimulus (fear) + Star of Bethlehem (trauma, shock).

This formula was administered in indirect application (20 drops in their trough).

The day after they started taking the remedies, Bony started approaching his new owner and he eventually completely recovered confidence. From then on, neither donkey tried to flee in panic every time someone tried to pet them, as they had done before treatment. Despite their rapid improvement we decided to continue the remedies for six more days.

Bony and Ruc are currently still living on the same farm where they were adopted and allow any member of the family to stroke them.

6.10.5 Fear and panic due to mistreatment

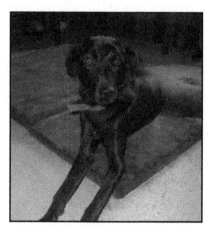

Name: Noa

Breed: Greyhound-labrador cross

Sex: Female

Age / Imprinting:
3½ years / unknown

Noa

Reason for consultation

Very extreme traumatic panic.

Noa was abandoned and run over by a car in a town in Lleida province (Spain). When she was rescued by volunteers from the Amics dels Animals de la Noguera shelter she was exhausted and badly injured. The tibia and fibula of one of her legs were broken in several places, she had bruises all over her body and was suffering from ehrlichiosis, an infectious disease caused by ticks. After successful surgery she was taken into a foster home. When she recovered she was admitted to the animal shelter. However, Noa's expression was of terror and she showed immense fear when approached, hardly interacting at all with the volunteers caring for her. She always had her tail between her legs and often sought a corner in which to hide. She did not interact with the other dogs either, except for her roommate.

Noa lived in a state of chronic stress, always on the alert, closely watching the movements of people around her. The traumatic panic that Noa experienced was so intense that she needed Flower treatment at a very high frequency. However, the animal shelter did not have the time required to apply the treatment at the necessary frequency.

Finally, we decided to adopt her ourselves and began to treat her with Flower Remedies.

Remedies administered orally

(Refer to 'Preparation of a remedy for oral application', p.21.)

> Rock Rose (panic) + Mimulus (fear) + Star of Bethlehem (trauma, shock) + Walnut (adaptation) + Olive (exhaustion).

The formula was administered at a rate of 4 drops, eight to ten times per day for one month, in direct application.

For the first 15 days, when we took Noa for a walk she stayed by our side constantly. If someone approached to stroke her, she would try to run away in the opposite direction, but was unable to do so because we always had her on a lead. If approached by another animal, she would bark to hold it off. At home she was always on the alert; during the day she would sleep little and could not relax. Most of the time she would scrutinize every move we made and hurried to hide under the table at the slightest noise. She accepted our stroking, but her body remained completely stiff. Gradually she began to accept other people's presence more positively, but not that of other dogs, except the two she lived with.

At the end of the first month of treatment she was not as alert when at home, although she was still very frightened whenever she saw the broom. She was not stiff any more when stroked; on the contrary, she even demanded to be petted. When walking in the street she began to accept the proximity of certain people, but did not let them touch her. She still held off any animals that got too close, using more force each time.

The formula that we administered to Noa for the first month was intended primarily to deal with the very evident after effects of traumatic panic, even though more than a year had passed since she was abandoned and run over by a car. We also added Olive to the formula, not because Noa was devitalized, but because she had lived for more than a year in a state of permanent stress, probably exhausting the kidney area.

To help Noa socialize with other animals in the neighbourhood we decided to add two remedies included in the fear-induced aggressiveness formula. Noa's new formula was as follows:

Rock Rose (panic) + Mimulus (fear) + Star of Bethlehem (trauma, shock) + Walnut (adaptation) + Olive (exhaustion) + Holly (mistrust) + Beech (intolerance).

It was administered at a rate of 4 drops, six times per day, in direct application, for three months.

After 15 days of treatment with this second formula, Noa would let some small dogs approach her in the street, still holding off the bigger dogs. During the three months of taking this formula, Noa gradually started socializing with people and other animals. At home she was perfectly adapted and became a very affectionate dog, but hid when she heard noises she did not recognize.

We decided to continue treatment with the same formula except for adding Chestnut Bud (learning process) instead of Walnut for three months at a rate of 4 drops, four times per day, in direct application.

Since the end of this period Noa has interacted with most small and medium-sized (her own size) dogs on the street and approaches people stroking other animals. She actually moves in front of them and waits to be petted.

Observations
Noa continues with the same treatment to this day.

6.10.6 Fear and panic: paralysis of bowel and sphincters

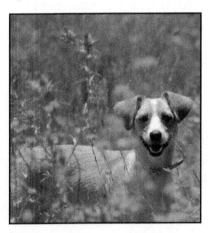

Laia

Name: Laia

Breed: Mixed

Sex: Female

Age / Imprinting:
2 years / unknown

Reason for consultation
Paralysis of bowel and sphincters.

Laia was found in the middle of some crop fields and was taken to the Amics dels Animals de la Noguera shelter. After ten days she was adopted and exchanged her peaceful refuge in a rural area for a home located in a city full of people and traffic. Although she seemed calm and happy, she did not urinate or defecate for the first 36 hours after she arrived in the big city, even though her new owners often took her out for walks. Probably as a result of the house move, Laia was frightened but did not express it through her behaviour.

REMEDIES ADMINISTERED ORALLY

A formula was prepared using the Rock Rose remedy (paralysis) and 4 drops were administered directly into her mouth. She was then taken for a walk, and within one minute Laia had defecated and urinated.

Remember that fear and/or panic can paralyze an organ or any motor activity of the body. In Laia's case, Rock Rose helped restore the peristaltic motility of her intestines (see Rock Rose, p.78).

6.10.7 Fear and panic: stroke

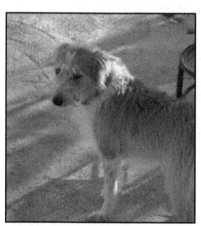

Name: Rufo

Breed: Mixed

Sex: Male

Age / Imprinting: 4 years / unknown

Rufo

Reason for consultation

Stroke.

Rufo arrived at Amics dels Animals de la Noguera animal shelter after being rescued by fire-fighters. He had been thrown down a 2.5-metre-deep sealed well with his legs tied up. Within a few days of his arrival at the animal shelter, he had a stroke and his legs were paralyzed. To rule out a spinal problem, he underwent a myelogram (a test that detects abnormalities in the spine, spinal cord or the surrounding areas) at Bellaterra Veterinary Hospital.

Animals that experience traumatic panic often suffer after effects that may later trigger the paralysis of an organ, limb or any other part of the body.

Remedies administered orally

(Refer to 'Preparation of a remedy for oral application', p.21.)

> Rock Rose (panic, paralysis) + Star of Bethlehem (trauma, shock).

Rufo did not receive a Flower treatment, but had he been given a preventive treatment soon after being rescued he may well have completely avoided post-traumatic secondary effects such as paralysis. The formula should have been administered at a rate of 4 drops, eight times per day, in direct application for a minimum of one week.

Rufo is now fully recovered, running and jumping on the paths surrounding the Amics dels Animals de la Noguera animal shelter, waiting to find a family to adopt him.

6.10.8 Fear and panic: facial paralysis

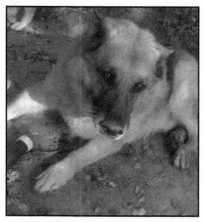

Zack

Name: Zack

Breed: German shepherd

Sex: Female

Age / Imprinting:
12 years / yes

REASON FOR CONSULTATION

Facial paralysis without any apparent cause.

Zack's face was paralyzed on the left side. The vet could find no cause to explain the sudden paralysis.

REMEDIES ADMINISTERED ORALLY

(Refer to 'Preparation of a remedy for oral application', p.21.)

> Mimulus (fear) + Rock Rose (paralysis) + Star of Bethlehem (trauma, shock) + Clematis (disconnection).

The formula was administered at a rate of 4 drops, four times per day, in direct application.

Remedies applied locally

> Mimulus (fear) + Rock Rose (paralysis) + Star of Bethlehem (trauma, shock) + Clematis (disconnection) + Hornbeam (laxity).

An oral preparation was made with the above formula. A sterile gauze was then impregnated with about 10 drops of the preparation. The gauze was then applied over the paralyzed area, allowing the remedies to take effect for at least one minute. This procedure was repeated several times a day depending on Zack's owner's time availability.

After one month of a combination of oral and local treatment, the paralyzed area of the left side of Zack's face started to move, thereby ending the treatment.

6.10.9 Fear and panic, emotional blockage

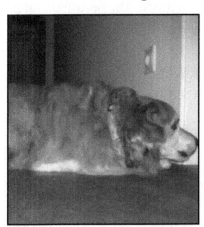

Name: Andreu

Breed: Mixed

Sex: Male

Age / Imprinting: 12 years / unknown

Andreu

Reason for consultation

Panic and refusal to go for a walk since the day his sister/companion had to be put down.

Andreu and Nora were born in the same litter and lived together for ten years. They got on very well and were always together. When Nora left the house to go outside, Andreu always went with her. Nora became very ill and finally had to be put down by the vet.

The day after Nora died, Andreu refused to go out when his owner showed him the lead and he had to be forced to go outside to urinate and defecate. From then on, Andreu did not want to go out and his owners had to force him to. At home he was calm but a little sad. After 15 days had passed Andreu's emotional situation had not improved and so his owners decided to start a Flower treatment.

Remedies administered orally

(Refer to 'Preparation of a remedy for oral application', p.21.)

> Mimulus (fear) + Rock Rose (panic) + Star of Bethlehem (shock, trauma) + Walnut (adaptation) + Honeysuckle (melancholy).

The formula was administered at a rate of 4 drops, four times per day, in direct application.

Within one week Andreu's behaviour had improved. He went outside without resistance, although he did not walk very far. As soon as he had urinated and defecated he immediately wanted to go home. After one month Andreu's emotional state had improved completely. Despite this, we decided to continue the treatment for one more month.

6.11 Pseudocyesis (psychological pregnancy)

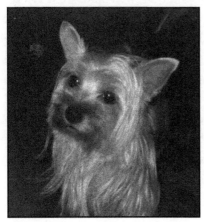

Name: Beky

Breed: Yorkshire

Sex: Female

Age / Imprinting:
5 years / unknown

Beky

Reason for consultation

Repeated pseudopregnancies.

Beky is a little female dog that always demanded a lot of attention from her owners. She often suffered pseudopregnancy (see 'Pseudocyesis/psychological pregnancy', p.130). She would become very sensitive, increasingly needing to be paid attention by her owners, demanding constant attention day and night. She whined all day and adopted a doll as her puppy, always covering it up with her sleeping blanket, but not becoming aggressive if it was removed. During the psychological pregnancy she also lost her appetite and lost weight.

REMEDIES ADMINISTERED ORALLY

(Refer to 'Preparation of a remedy for oral application', p.21.)

> Chicory (possessiveness) + Heather (demanding attention) + Holly (hypersensitivity) + Red Chestnut (detachment) + Walnut (adaptation to change) + Chestnut Bud (learning process).

The formula was administered at a rate of 4 drops, five times per day, in direct application.

After five days all of Beky's psychological pregnancy symptoms had stopped, but despite Beky's rapid improvement we decided to extend her treatment for one more month.

Psychological pregnancy usually occurs between a month and a half and two months after the female is in heat. As a preventive measure we therefore decided to treat Beky with this formula for ten days at a rate of 4 drops, four times per day, for about a month and a half after Beky stopped being in heat.

6.12 Feline urological syndrome (FUS)

How Bach Flowers can help an animal during the process of this disease

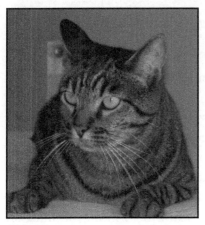

Name: Patxi

Breed: Domestic shorthaired

Sex: Male

Age / Imprinting:
5 years / unknown

Patxi

REASON FOR CONSULTATION

Feline urological syndrome.[1]

Due to the negligence of an airline company, Patxi had strayed into the area surrounding the airport as he was being prepared for transport abroad. He was adopted a few months later. One year

---

1 FUS includes several diseases of the cat's urinary tract which cause irritation of the mucous membrane lining the inside of the bladder and urethra. These diseases cause the various clinical signs that characterize this syndrome (difficulty urinating, blood in the urine and in some cases even total blockage). Cats affected by this disease frequently urinate small amounts and often do so outside the litter tray. Some cats also meow due to pain when urinating or when attempting to do so repeatedly and without success. Male cats tend to lick their penis. If the urinary tract is completely blocked, the animal will be dehydrated, depressed and may even vomit. Diet is among the many factors that may predispose a cat to suffer a urological syndrome.

Cats with an obstructed urinary tract will die if the urine flow is not restored within two to four days following the blockage. The reason for this is that complete blockage causes acute kidney failure which makes the kidneys stop filtering. Toxic waste then builds up in the blood causing heart and metabolic disorders, encephalopathies, etc., that cause the animal to die from shock.

after the airport incident he started vomiting repeatedly and the vet diagnosed feline urological syndrome.

Patxi's blood was analyzed and the urea and creatinine levels were found to be very high, confirming kidney malfunction. After a few days Patxi began to experience continuous urine loss and stopped eating, causing weight loss. His antibiotic treatment was changed several times, but Patxi did not recover. He only improved slightly when administered subcutaneous injected serum. A month and a half later, new analysis confirmed that although urea levels had decreased slightly since the first blood test, they were still very high. Patxi suffered from anaemia and his leukocyte levels were 89,000 (normal level is between 5500 and 19,500). He had lost two kilos (4½ lb) and had to be forced to eat. He was in a very deteriorated and apathetic state. Valium was injected intravenously but his emotional state did not improve. The vet decided to carry out tests for leukaemia, as his symptoms were similar to the ones characteristic of this disease, but the results came out negative.

Patxi's owner consulted another vet who recommended a change of antibiotic and to start a treatment to address the cat's emotional situation. At this point the owner decided to treat Patxi with Bach Flowers.

Remedies administered orally
(Refer to 'Preparation of a remedy for oral application', p.21.)

> Rock Rose (panic) + Star of Bethlehem (trauma, shock) + Olive (exhaustion, devitalization) + Elm (overwhelmed) + Sweet Chestnut (extreme anguish).

The formula was administered at a rate of 4 drops, four times per day, in direct application.

Two weeks after starting treatment Patxi had begun to wash himself, show an interest in the objects around him and climb and jump as normal, but did not recover his appetite. He lost another kilo in weight. We decided to continue with the same formula and increased the dosage rate from five to six times per day depending on the owner's availability. One week later a new blood test was carried out. The anaemia had disappeared and the leukocytes had decreased to 37,000, a level which was still too high, but this time Patxi had only lost 100 grams (4 oz) in weight. We decided to continue with the same treatment at the same rate for several more weeks. At the same time, the owner started colour therapy to improve the cat's renal area (kidney and adrenal glands), placing lilac and scarlet-coloured objects close by.

After two months of Flower treatment Patxi recovered some of his appetite and his emotional state returned to normal. An ultrasound scan confirmed that his kidneys had improved although one of them continued to be swollen. The vet believed the problems could become chronic. We decided to continue with the same formula and await progress.

After four months Patxi had fully recovered emotionally. The state of his kidneys was still delicate but they returned to the normal size, at which point the treatment was stopped.

6.13 Repetitive cough and early stage anaemia

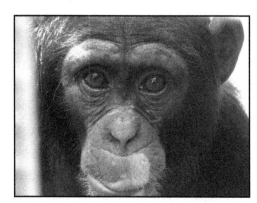

Name: Nita

Sex: Female (chimpanzee)

Age / Imprinting: 4 years / unknown

Nita

Case treated by Laura Riera (SEDIBAC (Society for the Study and Promotion of Bach Flower Remedies in Catalonia) volunteer) in the Tacugama Sanctuary (Sierra Leone) with the collaboration of the SEDIBAC animal volunteer team.

REASON FOR CONSULTATION

Chronic repetitive cough.

Nita was orphaned when a hunter killed her mother and probably other members of her family. She was later sold as a pet, and when she was one year old she arrived at Tacaguma sanctuary where she now lives with ten other chimpanzees aged between 4 and 12 years.

When she arrived at Tacugama, she was suspected of having tuberculosis and was isolated in quarantine during veterinary tests. During this period Bach Flower Therapy was the only treatment given.

Remedies administered orally
(Refer to 'Preparation of a remedy for oral application', p.21.)

> Crab Apple (cleanse) + Gorse (for its positive effect on the immune system) + Walnut (adaptation) + Olive (exhaustion and lack of vitality) + Centaury (weakness) + White Chestnut (repetition).

The formula was administered at a rate of 4 drops, 10–12 times per day, in direct application.

On the first day of treatment Nita began to cough less, and by the second day the coughing was considerably reduced. On the fifth day the coughing ceased completely, but she was apathetic, manifesting a state of despondency. Gentian was added to the previous formula and treatment was continued for three more days.

After a total of eight days of treatment, Nita didn't cough any more and started being a little more cheerful. We decided to end the treatment and await the results of the tuberculosis test.

Observations
The tests ruled out tuberculosis and revealed early anaemia. This was treated according to the criteria of the centre's veterinarian.

7

A SELECTION OF CASES TREATED BY LOCAL APPLICATION

7.1 Allergies

Name: Sky

Breed: Labrador

Sex: Male

Age / Imprinting: 2 years / yes

REASON FOR CONSULTATION

Acute allergy in the neck area to the active ingredient of anti-parasite pipettes.

Sky's allergy manifested as inflammation, pain when touched, severe irritation of the affected area and scabs. Anti-inflammatory drugs did not improve the situation and neither did cortisone. The allergy became more and more acute and was accompanied by recurrent infections that do not respond to antibiotic treatment.

Remedies administered as a cream

(Refer to 'Preparation of a Flower cream', p.23.)

> Rescue Remedy (physical shock due to intoxication) + Crab Apple (cleanse) + Agrimony (agonizing itch) + Beech (irritation) + Vervain (inflammation).

Treatment

After one week of treatment (three daily applications) the scab had disappeared and the area had completely regenerated.

7.2 Pus lumps

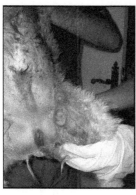
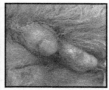
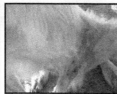

Name: Pipin

Breed: Mixed

Sex: Male

Age / Imprinting:
3 years / unknown

Pipin (detail)

REASON FOR CONSULTATION

Swollen and infected cutaneous lumps with secretion of pus and abundant liquid matter in the interior. Considerable pain, sensitive to touch.

The vet performed surgery to open one of the lumps, and confirmed the presence of grass seeds inside. Together we assessed the application of a Flower Remedy cream over the lumps and for the time being ruled out any further surgery.

REMEDIES ADMINISTERED AS A CREAM

(Refer to 'Preparation of a Flower cream', p.23.)

> Crab Apple (cleanse) + Elm (pain sensitive to touch) + Vervain (inflammation) + Vine (liquid causing pressure, pus).

TREATMENT

Twenty-four hours later (four topical applications) one of the lumps exploded; there was a large discharge of pus and the grass seed surfaced. The grass seed was extracted with some sterilized tweezers and we continued to apply the cream to all the lumps (two daily applications). The problem was resolved in three weeks.

7.3 Conjunctivitis

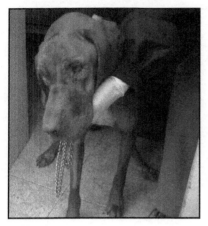

Name: Misia

Breed: Mixed

Sex: Female

Age / Imprinting:
3 years / unknown

Misia

REASON FOR CONSULTATION

Swollen cutaneous lumps. Infectious conjunctivitis.

Misia was found in deplorable conditions, very malnourished, with the skin of her abdominal area irritated and open and the area surrounding her eyes red and swollen. She also presented infectious conjunctivitis and was in heat. The vet certified that she had been poisoned and that she was very malnourished. After being admitted to a veterinary clinic for several days, she entered the Amics dels Animals de la Noguera shelter. As well as presenting a general state of panic, her face expressed desolation, exhaustion and great sadness.

Remedies administered as eye-drops
(Refer to 'Preparation of Flower eye-drops', p.24.)

> Beech (irritation) + Crab Apple (cleanse) + Olive (lack of vitality) + Vervain (inflammation).

Treatment

With sterile saline solution and the above-mentioned remedies, we prepared eye-drops and applied 2 drops in each eye, three times per day. After each application, a few drops were poured on a sterile gauze and placed for a few seconds on the area around the eyes.

A Flower Remedy cream was also applied in the abdominal area in order to deal with the after effects of the poison that oozed through her abdomen (see Case 7.7, p.204).

Simultaneously with the topical treatments, Misia was treated with an oral preparation in order to deal with her despondency, sadness and remnants of traumatic panic (see Case 6.10.3, p.175).

After eight days, Misia's appearance had completely changed: her abdominal area and the outline of her eyes were no longer red and showed no signs of irritation. Her physical condition improved considerably, she gained weight and the infectious conjunctivitis also remitted, but she still expressed sadness and fear.

Oral treatment was continued for three weeks. After this time, Misia was adopted and her new family informed us that she had adapted very easily to her new home.

7.4 Infection and abscess of the anal glands

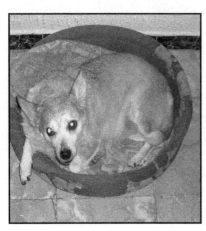

Name: Chispa

Breed: Mixed

Sex: Female

Age / Imprinting:
11 years / unknown

Chispa

REASON FOR CONSULTATION

Swollen skin lumps. Infection and obstruction of the anal glands (anal sacs).

Chispa was an old dog that presented with an abscess: a swelling which was warm and when broken discharged blood and pus. She developed a fistula as a result of infection of the anal glands.

The anal glands or sacs are two pouches located on either side of the anus. Normally these glands are emptied during defecation. Sometimes they are not, and their content becomes denser, making it more difficult to empty them. This situation is called impaction, and to resolve it the dog usually adopts the characteristic posture of sitting on its back paws and dragging its anus on the floor while moving slowly. This soothes itching and pain in the anal area. Impaction may be complicated by an infection that manifests as fever with some haemorrhaging. If the infection is not treated rapidly, an abscess can form, which usually requires surgical intervention.

Remedies administered as a cream
(Refer to 'Preparation of a Flower cream', p.23.)

Crab Apple (cleanse) + Star of Bethlehem (scarring) + Vervain (inflammation) + Walnut (cut, blood-clotting).

Treatment

Due to Chispa's weight and old age, her owner did not want to risk surgery. We decided to prepare a cream, and a sterile gauze was soaked in it and then held for at least one minute on the anal area. We used a sterile gauze instead of directly applying the cream in order to make sure that the cream was in contact with the anus for the minimum amount of time needed to be effective. When the cream was applied directly, Chispa would lick the area constantly. Given the fact that she had easy access to the treated area, we decided to make four applications per day instead of two to three, which is the usual procedure. After ten days the anal glands stopped seeping blood. Despite this, a preventive treatment was continued for two months, applying the cream with a gauze two times per day. Chispa's anal glands have not bled any more and we were able to avoid surgery.

Observations

Prior to local treatment with Bach Flower Remedies, Chispa had received oral treatment with antibiotics and a stomach protector, and a cream with anti-inflammatory, anti-pruritic and vasoconstrictor properties was applied locally. These treatments failed to definitively resolve the infection and inflammation of the anal glands. When receiving medical treatment Chispa improved and her anal problem remitted, but after a few weeks she would suffer a relapse, even if the vet had manually cleansed her anal glands.

7.5 Inflammation and infection of the third eyelid

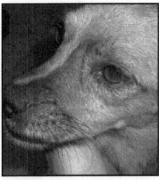

Name: Lluna

Breed: Mixed

Sex: Female

Age / Imprinting:
7 years / unknown

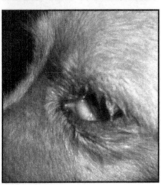

Lluna

Reason for consultation

Inflammation and infection of the third eyelid.

Lluna presented recurrent infections and inflammations of the third eyelid.

The third eyelid produces tears and protects the eye from external aggressions. All animals have this additional protection, which must be carefully preserved as it carries out very important functions. If the third eyelid remains over the eye for longer than usual this may indicate the presence of infections, lesions over the ocular globe, ulcers and wounds.

Remedies administered as eye-drops
(Refer to 'Preparation of Flower eye-drops', p.24.)

> Crab Apple (cleanse) + Beech (irritation) + Vervain (inflammation) + Holly (rage).

We decided to include Holly (rage) in the formula because it is a negative characteristic of Lluna's character and, moreover, because the third eyelid would suddenly and abruptly flick out from under her eyelid.

Treatment

Two drops of the eye-drop preparation were applied to the affected eye, four times per day. Over the following 48 hours the infection disappeared and the third eyelid returned to its original position. In spite of this quick improvement, treatment was continued for ten more days, applying the eye-drops only two times per day.

Observations

In the beginning an eye-drop preparation was prepared with the three first remedies, but only the infection remitted and swelling of the third eyelid continued. The problem was not completely solved until Holly (rage) was added to the formula.

Lluna has presented this problem again every time that a new animal has entered her home, but in all cases, the third eyelid has swollen without becoming infected with no further treatment required.

7.6 Leishmaniasis

How Bach Flowers can help in the treatment of the cutaneous conditions of an animal with Leishmaniasis

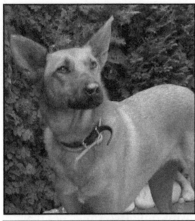
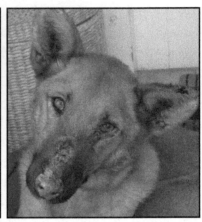
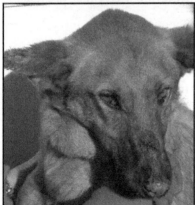

Name: Nyolis

Breed: Mixed

Sex: Female

Age / Imprinting:
5 years / unknown

Nyolis

REASON FOR CONSULTATION

Skin lesions due to Leishmaniasis: alopecia, necrosis, scabbing and ulceration (see also Leishmaniasis, p.166).

Leishmaniasis is a disease caused by a parasite that invades different organs of the dog, causing injuries of varying gravity and eventually causing the animal's death. A mosquito called phlebotomus transmits this parasite to the dog through its bite.

Clinical symptomatology is very diverse, but the following are some examples: skin lesions (alopecia, scabbing, ulcers), lesions in the joints, weight loss, muscle atrophy, haemorrhages, increase in size of liver and spleen, limping and, when the disease is in an advanced state, signs of kidney failure. Ulcers are mainly located on different parts of the head (snout, ears, around the eyes, etc.).

Remedies administered as a cream with Aloe Vera

(Refer to 'Preparation of a Flower cream', p.23.)

> Beech (irritation) + Crab Apple (cleanse) + Star of Bethlehem (traumatism) + Hornbeam (local energy) + Olive (revitalizing) + Centaury (weakness) + Clematis (disconnection).

Treatment

Aloe Vera is used as the diluent vehicle because sometimes when Flower Remedies are applied in a neutral cream base the treated area becomes even more reddened. The affected areas were treated three times per day for 15 days. The skin ulcerations healed, reducing irritation and redness in the area. Treatment was continued for two more weeks. After one month, alopecia and scabbing had disappeared.

Observations

The last four remedies in the formula are energy contributors. In most skin problems Olive + Hornbeam are used, but in Leishmaniasis, being a disease of infectious aetiology, the animal must overcome the characteristics of the disease without giving in, and reconnect the energy flow in the necrosed areas.

7.7 Sores and burns as a result of poisoning

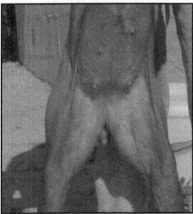

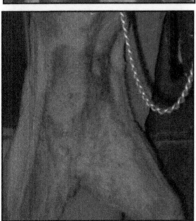

Misia (detail)

Name: Misia

Breed: Mixed

Sex: Female

Age / Imprinting:
3 years / unknown

REASON FOR CONSULTATION

Sores and burns on the skin.

Misia was found in deplorable conditions: she was very malnourished, the skin on her abdomen was irritated and very raw, and the area around her eyes was red and swollen. She also presented infectious conjunctivitis (see Case 7.3, p.196) and was in heat. The vet certified that she had been poisoned and was rather malnourished. After being hospitalized for several days in a veterinary clinic, she entered the Amics dels Animals de la Noguera animal shelter where she was treated with vitamin supplements and Bach Flower Remedies.

Besides being in a general state of panic, her face expressed despair, exhaustion and great sadness.

Remedies administered as a cream

(Refer to 'Preparation of a Flower cream', p.23.)

> Crab Apple (cleanse) + Beech (irritation) + Holly (rash) + Olive (revitalizing) + Star of Bethlehem (traumatism) + Vervain (inflammation).

Treatment

The Flower Remedy cream was applied two times per day to deal with the after effects of the poison that coursed through her irritated, red abdomen. At the same time, eye-drops and oral remedies were applied to treat dejection, sadness and the after effects of traumatic panic that she manifested when she arrived at the animal shelter (see Case 6.10.3, p.175).

Eight days later, Misia's appearance had completely changed; her abdominal area and the outline of her eyes were no longer red and showed no signs of irritation. Her physical condition had improved considerably, she had gained weight, and the infectious conjunctivitis had also remitted. However, Misia still expressed sadness and fear.

Oral treatment was maintained for three more weeks. After this time, she was adopted and her new family informed us that she had adapted very easily to her new home.

7.8 Mastitis

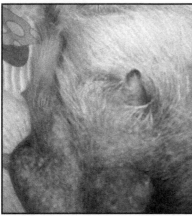

Name: Wilma

Breed: Labrador

Sex: Female

Age / Imprinting:
6 years / unknown

Wilma (detail)

REASON FOR CONSULTATION

Inflammation of the mammary glands after giving birth.

Wilma rejected her puppies out of jealousy and even bit off a piece of one of the puppies' ears (see Case 6.3.1, p.154). Wilma eventually recovered from her jealousy and returned to nursing her puppies. Approximately one month after nursing, Wilma suffered from mastitis.

REMEDIES ADMINISTERED AS A CREAM

(Refer to 'Preparation of a Flower cream', p.23.)

> Beech (irritation) + Crab Apple (cleanse) + Holly (rash) + Star of Bethlehem (traumatism) + Vervain (inflammation).

TREATMENT

A cream was applied three times per day to each of the red, swollen glands. After one week, the mastitis had improved considerably. We decided to continue with local treatment for one more week.

OBSERVATIONS

Although treatment for swelling and redness of the mammary glands was carried out with Vervain, we decided to add Holly (jealousy) to the cream because the mammary area was hot and Wilma expressed jealousy every time her owner petted the puppies.

7.9 Cutaneous nodule of unknown aetiology

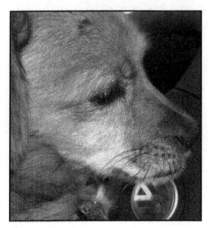

Name: Lluna

Breed: Mixed

Sex: Female

Age / Imprinting:
7 years / unknown

Lluna

REASON FOR CONSULTATION

Rapidly growing cutaneous nodule with a similar size and shape to a lentil, black in colour, with a very hard texture. Not painful when touched. It was very localized and the area around it showed no inflammation.

REMEDIES ADMINISTERED AS A CREAM

(Refer to 'Preparation of a Flower cream', p.23.)

> Chicory (retention) + Crab Apple (cleanse) + Rock Water (hardness) + Vine (liquid causing pressure).

Treatment

The cream was applied in the morning and evening for 15 days. The nodule stopped growing but maintained its original appearance, texture and size. After 20 days of treatment, its size began to diminish rapidly, and on the 21st day the nodule was completely reabsorbed.

Observations

One of the transpersonal applications of the Chicory remedy is to manage retained accumulations (including liquids such as water or blood, fat or faeces). In this case Vine, which follows the pattern of fluid pressure, acted synergistically with Chicory to release the content of the nodule and dispose of it safely into the bloodstream.

7.10 Traumatism

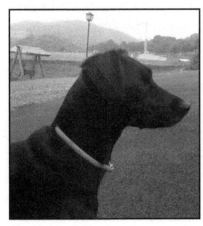

Name: Noa

Breed: Greyhound-Labrador cross

Sex: Female

Age / Imprinting:
4 years / unknown

Noa

Reason for consultation

Traumatism caused by a fall. Limping on one leg.

While running through the mountains, Noa jumped from a height of about two metres. When she reached the ground she began walking with the leg tucked up, not letting it touch the ground. She stopped often and soon after she refused to walk. When any part of her leg was touched she didn't complain, nor when we manually moved her joints. We also confirmed that there was nothing embedded in any area of the affected foot.

Even after resting for four hours she still walked with the leg tucked up without it touching the ground. At first glance, there was no inflammation visible to the naked eye. We decided to prepare a cream with Bach Flowers.

Remedies administered as a cream

(Refer to 'Preparation of a Flower cream', p.23).

> Hornbeam (specific weakness) + Elm (overwhelmed due to overload of any type) + Star of Bethlehem (traumatism).

Treatment

In the absence of pain, sensitivity to touch or swelling, we were not sure what area of the leg was affected. We therefore decided to apply cream every half hour to the whole leg and carpal area, performing a gentle massage until the cream was absorbed (approximately one minute). The massage was intended to divert the animal's attention and prevent her from licking her leg immediately after each application.

After the fourth application Noa's limp disappeared.

Observations

Although the animal did not feel any pain when palpated, we decided to administer Elm because we interpreted that the traumatism had been caused by an overload in one area of the leg when it hit the ground. Elm would also give energy to her muscles.

8

WORK METHODOLOGY FOR ANIMAL SHELTERS

Formulas and Guidelines

There are currently many animal shelters that have neither the staff nor the necessary time to treat each animal that manifests an anomalous behaviour. The animals at a shelter are often scared or depressed because they have been mistreated and/or abandoned prior to their admission to the shelter. They may also show some aggressiveness due to territoriality or fear. The increasing number of abandoned animals and animal shelters' lack of economic resources to enlarge kennel facilities create space issues which may lead to aggressiveness in animals living together in the same area. Thus, it has become necessary for us to prioritize the use of Flower Remedies, limiting oral and local remedy application to only the animals that are arriving at shelters and those that are leaving into foster care or adoption.

Most of the animals that have just joined the shelter are given the appropriate formula for 15 days at a rate of 4 drops, four times per day. Normally, the duration of the treatment should be at least of one month and it would be advisable to continue with it for two to five months depending on the intensity of the problem being treated. However, the lack of both volunteers and time may prevent shelters from following the recommended duration and frequency of the treatment. This partly explains the differences observed in the effectiveness of formulas in newly arrived animals. Effectiveness also depends on whether the animal remains in the shelter or goes within a few days to either a foster home or into adoption where its problems may be treated in depth, allowing its treatment to have the appropriate duration and frequency. In addition, whenever circumstances allow, we recommend increasing the frequency of the treatment to six times per day during the first week.

Treatments addressed to recently arrived animals

Animals that don't manifest any behavioural problem

Usually these are animals that have been lost or abandoned with no microchip[1] or ID tag.[2] In order to facilitate their adaptation to the conditions of the shelter (new territory, living with other animals, etc.) administer the following formula for a minimum of 15 days at a rate of 4 drops, four times per day (see 'Preparation of a remedy for oral application', p.21):

> Beech (intolerance) + Holly (jealousy, possible aggressiveness) + Star of Bethlehem (trauma) + Rock Rose (panic) + Walnut (adaptation).

When you have no knowledge of the animal's past, the intake of Rock Rose and Star of Bethlehem is essential as these remedies deal with the after effects of a possible shock or post-traumatic stress.

---

1   By European Union law it is obligatory for all pet owners to install a microchip in their animals to facilitate their identification. When an animal is placed under the microchip reader, the microchip provides all the details on the animal and its owner. This system has two advantages: first, a lost animal can be reunited with its owner, and second, owners who abandon animals can be held accountable.

2   This tag has the name and telephone number of the owner for the animal's quick and easy identification.

Sometimes these after effects manifest as sudden illness (paralysis, stroke, etc.). Walnut is added to the formula in order to foster the animal's adaptability to its new situation, and Holly and Beech in order to facilitate coexistence with other animals, especially with regards to sharing food and space.

Animals that manifest fear, panic and/or hyperventilation when arriving at the shelter

For animals of a timid and fearful nature, and those that manifest fear when facing their new circumstances, administer the following formula for at least 15 days at a rate of 4 drops, four times per day (see 'Preparation of a remedy for oral application', p.21):

> Beech (intolerance) + Holly (jealousy, possible aggressiveness) + Star of Bethlehem (trauma) + Walnut (adaptation) + Rock Rose (panic) + Sweet Chestnut (anguish) + Rescue Remedy (if the animal is very restless).

The first four remedies, common to the previous formula, make it easy for the animal to adapt to its new situation. The last three help manage the fear, worry and anxiety that its new circumstances imply and also 'cleanse' the residues of distressing panic from its past. Furthermore, especially if the animal hyperventilates, Rock Rose will help release tension caused by the stress experienced in the period between abandonment and rescue. In very acute cases also consider adding Rescue Remedy.

The last three remedies of the formula are also widely used in animals that experience extreme stress when confronted with loud noises such as thunder, fireworks, festivals, fairs, celebrations, etc.

Animals that manifest fear or panic due to mistreatment and show signs of malnutrition

If the animal arriving at the shelter is scared and thin with clear signs of malnutrition, after the vet has ruled out illness, administer the following formula for a minimum of 15 days at a rate of 4 drops, six times per day during the first week. After that first week, administer it at a rate of 4 drops, four times per day (see 'Preparation of a remedy for oral application', p.21):

Star of Bethlehem (trauma) + Walnut (adaptation) + Rock Rose (panic) + Sweet Chestnut (anguish) + Olive (exhaustion).

Olive is administered to an animal which is exhausted due to a previous situation of suffering, including malnutrition due to abandonment, devitalization, being run over by a car, attempted poisoning, mistreatment, etc. Star of Bethlehem, Rock Rose and Sweet Chestnut will help it deal with the after effects of panic and anguish as a result of the traumatic situation it experienced. Moreover, Walnut will enable it to adapt better to its new circumstances.

If the animal arrives dying of starvation, not of disease, add Gorse (submission) to the above formula. Also add it if the animal refuses to eat not because of a physiological disease but because it has given up fighting for survival. The joint action of Olive and Gorse enhances the correct functioning of its immune system.

Animals that manifest certain types of aggressiveness

If an animal that arrives at the shelter has some type of aggressiveness, be it towards the staff or other animals, administer the following formula for a minimum of 15 days at a rate of 4 drops, six times per day for the first week and then decrease the dose to 4 drops, four times per day (see 'Preparation of a remedy for oral application', p.21):

Beech (intolerance) + Holly (jealousy, aggressiveness) + Star of Bethlehem (trauma) + Walnut (adaptation) + Cherry

Plum (loss of control) + Vine (domination) + Rock Rose (panic).

For cats you should also add Willow (resentment).

The first four remedies help the animal to adapt to its new environment. Vine is added to help with territorial or domination aggression, Rock Rose is for fear-induced aggression, and Cherry Plum helps an animal that seems calm and affectionate but suddenly attacks without reason.

Willow, together with Beech, is very useful for cats, the latter being the characteristic remedy of many of them. The combination of these two remedies helps the cat tolerate change better.

If in any of the above-mentioned situations the animal's behavioural problem persists for longer than two weeks, we recommend adding Rock Water (resistance to change) and Chestnut Bud (learning process) to the formula.

Treatments for animals leaving the shelter for adoption or foster care

SEDIBAC (the Society for the Study and Promotion of Bach Flower Therapy in Catalonia) currently offers a free service to people fostering or adopting an animal from the Amics dels Animals de la Noguera shelter (www.amicsdelsanimalsdelanoguera.org). This service covers assessment, treatment and monitoring of the behavioural problems manifested by the adopted or fostered animal and the animals that will live with it.

The primary goals of this free service are to investigate and spread the application of Bach Flowers to animals and to help resolve the behavioural patterns that hinder the animal's coexistence with its new family, which in many cases cause the animal's return to the shelter. These returns significantly worsen both the animals' emotional health and the economic situation of many shelters.

When addressing a specific behavioural problem, treatment applied to adopted or fostered animals is more successful than treatment applied to animals living in shelters. The reason for this is obvious: the former receive longer, more continuous treatment than the latter.

Animals that have not manifested any behavioural problem during their stay at the animal shelter

Even if an animal has adapted well to the shelter and has not manifested any anomalous behaviour during its stay, it is important that it leaves the shelter with a treatment focused on adapting to its new circumstances (new home, new family, coexistence with other animals, etc.).

It is recommended that the following formula be used for a minimum of 15 days at a rate of 4 drops, four times per day (see 'Preparation of a remedy for oral application', p.21).

> Chicory (possessiveness) + Heather (demanding attention) + Star of Bethlehem (trauma) + Walnut (adaptation) + Rock Rose (panic).

After two weeks, and depending on how the animal reacts, the need to continue the treatment or start a different one should be evaluated. Remember that we are dealing with animals with a history of abandonment and mistreatment. Although the change of habitat is positive for most of them, some may experience it as a traumatic situation, as it is once again leaving behind its environment, its companions, its carers, and so on. Rock Rose and Star of Bethlehem help to manage the potential traumas and phobias associated with the change of situation, Walnut will make adaptation easier, and Chicory and Heather will help the animal to avoid establishing an excessively possessive connection with its new family. This type of connection is one of the factors that induces anxiety in the animal each time it is left alone at home (see 'Separation anxiety', p.111).

If the animal is fostered or adopted into a home where there are children and/or other animals you should add Holly (jealousy), Beech (intolerance) and Cherry Plum (lack of control) to the above formula and treat the animal for at least one month at a rate of 4 drops, five or six times per day. In these cases the formula is as follows:

> Chicory (possessiveness) + Heather (demanding attention) + Walnut (adaptation) + Rock Rose (panic) + Star of Bethlehem (trauma) + Beech (intolerance) + Cherry Plum (lack of control, hysteria) + Holly (jealousy).

It is important that an animal that will live with children and/or other animals quickly learns to share food, space, affection and attention. This prevents unnecessary 'returns' and other more serious problems. We have found that the remedies Chicory, Heather and Walnut are not always sufficient to harmonize the animal's coexistence with its new family. The addition of Holly and Beech deals effectively with a situation of jealousy and rejection towards another family member. Furthermore, Cherry Plum helps to control aggressive impulses when sharing food and toys, or when it has to be brushed and have wounds cleaned.

As a means of prevention and caution, it is advisable to apply the same formula to the animals already living with the adoptive or foster family.

If the animal has not adapted after two weeks of treatment, add Rock Water (resistance to change) and Chestnut Bud (learning process) to the formula.

Animals of a fearful type

This character type is described in Section 5.11.4, p.128. These animals should be treated with the following formula at a rate of 4 drops, six times per day for a period of three to six months (see 'Preparation of a remedy for oral application', p.21):

> Chicory (possessiveness) + Heather (demanding attention) + Star of Bethlehem (trauma) + Walnut (adaptation) + Rock Rose (panic) + Olive (exhaustion).

To treat animals of a fearful nature, and those that manifest signs of having experienced a traumatic event (an accident, mistreatment, etc.), Rock Rose should be added to the first four remedies of the above formula (this is often the case for an animal which is fostered or adopted).

Animals of a fearful nature, such as those that have suffered traumatic events, often live on the alert, even when they are in no imminent danger. When suffering is sustained the energy of the kidney area is weakened. Olive is therefore an important remedy for animals living under chronic stress.

Animal of a nervous and/or anxious type

This type of animal needs to be treated as soon as possible with a formula that lowers its anxiety level, at a rate of 4 drops, five to eight times per day depending on the intensity of symptoms (see 'Preparation of a remedy for oral application', p.21):

> Rescue Remedy (emergency) + Star of Bethlehem (trauma) + Walnut (adaptation) + Agrimony (anxiety) + Impatiens (acceleration) + Vervain (overexcitement) + White Chestnut (accelerated repetition).

Star of Bethlehem is also included in this formula because we are dealing with animals that have been abandoned, and Walnut will facilitate their adaptation. The other remedies are aimed at managing the animals' anxiety and nervous nature, also moderating their hyperactivity. In very nervous animals, Cherry Plum is also added to help them release their inner tension.

When the anxiety level improves, a customized formula is used which, as well as regulating the anxiety, also treats its cause. Rock Rose deals with the possible fear and insecurity underlying this anxiety and nervousness, Heather treats excessive demands for attention, and Chicory and Star of Bethlehem treat fear of being abandoned again.

Unsociable behaviour is observed in some puppies with this character type. When separated from their mother prematurely they have not experienced the whole socialization process (four months), a period when important codes and interaction with their siblings are learned. In these cases we also recommend adding Chestnut Bud (learning process) to the formula mentioned above.

Local treatments

The third treatment method corresponds to the local treatments which have proven very effective, especially for ocular and dermatological problems.

Eye-drops for dogs and cats with eye infection

A formula is prepared with a sterile saline solution and the remedies listed below (see 'Preparation of Flower eye-drops', p.24). Apply two drops in each eye, two to three times per day. If the ocular infection is acute, the treatment can be complemented by cleaning the exterior area of the eye with a sterile gauze soaked in an aqueous solution containing the same remedies as the eye-drops. Repeat this every time the drops are applied to the interior of the eye.

Two to three days' treatment will be enough for the infection to subside. Nevertheless, it is recommended that you carry on the treatment for five to seven more days.

> Beech (irritation) + Crab Apple (cleanse) + Vervain (inflammation).

Eye infections produce significant inflammation of the conjunctiva, which is treatable with Vervain. This inflammation consequently produces irritation of the interior area of the eye, hence the need to apply Beech. When inflammation and irritation are severe (i.e. the animal cannot stop scratching its eyes) also consider adding Agrimony or Holly, depending on the animal's character type. These remedies will help deal with the incessant itching. Finally, the action of Crab Apple will help to cleanse the infected area energetically.

Peripheral corneal ulcers

Prepare eye-drops with a sterile saline solution and the remedies listed below (see 'Preparation of Flower eye-drops', p.24). Apply a few drops of this formula on a sterile gauze, leaving this compress on the damaged ocular area for a few seconds, at least three times per day.

> Beech (irritation) + Crab Apple (cleanse) + Hornbeam (local energy) + Star of Bethlehem (cicatrizant) + Vervain (inflammation).

The eye-drops should also be prepared with a sterile saline solution even if the ulcers are on the outside of the eye. The periphery of the eye is a very sensitive area and if you use mineral water as the diluent vehicle for the remedies it is probable that the animal will feel pain and a burning sensation during each application.

In most cases the ulcers swell and irritate the surrounding area. Again, Vervain and Beech will be of great help to reduce inflammation and irritation. Usually the area is devitalized as a result of the small ulcers: Hornbeam will provide sufficient local energy to enhance the cicatrizant action of Star of Bethlehem. Both remedies work at a physical and a psycho-emotional level; Star of Bethlehem also repairs the wounds that result from a traumatic situation at an energetical level. The presence of an ulcer means that the tissue is torn, and this injury will be repaired by the cicatrizant action of Star of Bethlehem. Finally, Crab Apple will help to energetically cleanse the affected area (see Case 7.7, p.204).

Skin allergy to anti-parasite pipettes

Some animals are allergic to the components of anti-parasite pipettes. The area that is in contact with the pipette medication becomes swollen, irritated and red, often producing an infected ulcer that eventually has to be treated with antibiotics (see Case 7.1, p.193).

To solve this problem, prepare a cream using a neutral cream base or Aloe Vera gel (for its regenerative properties) and add the following remedies (see 'Preparation of a Flower cream', p.23) with at least two applications per day:

Rescue Remedy (physical shock due to poisoning) + Crab Apple (cleanse) + Agrimony (unbearable itching) + Beech (irritation) + Vervain (inflammation).

The joint action of Rescue Remedy and Crab Apple helps to cleanse the physical after effects of local intoxication (physical shock) caused by the components of the anti-parasite liquid.[3] The area that is in contact with the allergen is swollen and red, and the animal scratches itself continuously and desperately, hence the need to add Vervain to treat swelling and redness, Beech to treat local irritation due to intoxication and also the animal's scratching, and Agrimony because the level of itchiness is high as a result of the inflammation and irritation in the area.

Cream for lumps with pus secretion

These types of lumps are usually formed when a grass seed is caught in the animal's skin (while the animal is running through the crop fields). If it is not removed in time it will normally cause an infection and secrete pus.

---

3   After the death of Dr Bach, the Rescue Cream (Rescue Remedy + Crab Apple mixed in a neutral cream base) was commercialized. This combination is a local emergency remedy for any physical shock or stress.

To avoid surgical extraction of the grass seed, prepare a cream with a neutral cream base or Aloe Vera gel and add the remedies listed below (see 'Preparation of a Flower cream', p.23):

Crab Apple (cleanse) + Elm (pain sensitive to touch) + Vervain (inflammation) + Vine (liquid causing pressure: pus).

In any process of local infection it is necessary to help drain the material (pus) produced in the infected area. Vine, like a grape, is associated with a liquid causing pressure. This remedy encourages the rupture of the lump and the expulsion of the pus inside, and Crab Apple completes the cleansing of the area. Usually such an infection produces a severe swelling (treatable with Vervain) and a lot of pain (improved with the action of Elm).

This cream is applied to each lump at least three to four times per day. After a few applications the lump opens, exposing the grass seed that caused the infection, which is then easily removed using sterilized tweezers (see Case 7.2, p.195).

Once the lump has exploded, prepare another cream with Aloe Vera gel and the following remedies and apply at least twice per day:

Rescue Remedy (physical trauma due to rupture of tissue) + Crab Apple (cleanse) + Elm (pain sensitive to touch) + Vervain (inflammation).

Cream to treat necrosis of the peripheral area of the ear

One of the cutaneous conditions manifested by the animal with Leishmaniasis is necrosis of the peripheral area of the ears (see Case 7.6, p.202). If this problem is not treated locally, the necrotic area will increase in size and black scabs will appear in the peripheral area of the ears, causing hair loss in that area and decreasing the size of the animal's ear.

To solve this problem prepare a cream with Aloe Vera gel (for its regenerative properties) and add the remedies listed below (see 'Preparation of a Flower cream', p.23):

> Rescue Remedy (physical trauma due to rupture of tissue) + Crab Apple (cleanse) + Hornbeam (local energy) + Olive (revitalization) + Star of Bethlehem (energetical repair).

Apply in the areas with necrosis, at least three times per day.

The properties of the Rescue Cream (Rescue Remedy + Crab Apple) are enhanced by the action of Star of Bethlehem which treats the disconnection or energetic breakage of the necrotic area, by the action of Hornbeam for the energetic weakening of the area, and finally by the action of Olive that revitalizes this area due to its energetic input.

Specific guidelines for animal shelters

In animal shelters there are specific risk situations requiring mass treatment of all the animals. This is the case for kennel cough and colds in winter which occur due to low temperatures, especially in shelters located in rural areas.

For kennel cough, it is recommended that pharmacological treatment be complemented with Bach Flower Therapy. For colds, it is recommended that a preventive Bach Flower treatment be carried out for one month before winter arrives and throughout the winter period.

Kennel cough (canine infectious tracheobronchitis)

In Autumn 2007, 175 dogs suffered from kennel cough in one of the animal shelters where SEDIBAC volunteers.

What is kennel cough?

Its scientific name is 'canine infectious tracheobronchitis' and it only affects dogs. It is usually a mild respiratory disease except in the cases of very young or very old dogs.

The infection is caused by three types of viruses (Reovirus, Adenovirus type 2 and Parainfluenzavirus) and by one bacteria (Bordetella Bronchiseptica). It has an incubation period of about three to four days from the time the animal enters into contact with these microorganisms.

What are the symptoms?

The main symptom is a persistent dry cough that ends in a kind of retch. It sounds like the dog has a foreign object in its throat and is trying to expel it. As a result it usually vomits bile. If the animal is not treated, it stops eating. The cough can last for days or even weeks.

How is it spread?

Although it is a mild disease, it is very contagious and is transmitted by direct contact or proximity. To catch kennel cough, it is enough for the animal to breathe infected particles in the air or drink water contaminated with the microorganisms.

An animal can catch it anywhere: in the street, parks, veterinary clinics, boarding kennels, competitions and exhibitions. It is even possible to catch kennel cough in a building's lift if an infected dog has used the lift previously.

Pharmacological treatment

This should be carried out according to the criteria of the animal shelter's vet.

COMPLEMENTARY TREATMENT WITH BACH FLOWERS

It is recommended that pharmacological treatment be complemented by administering a Bach Flower formula to all dogs living in the animal shelter where the disease outbreak has occurred. This is also the case when any animals at home have the disease.

The formula quoted below is the formula that the canine trainer and Bach Flower Therapist Antonio Paramio (2009) presented in his 'Kennel cough' talk:

> Beech (irritation) + Centaury (submission) + Crab Apple (cleanse) + Vervain (inflammation) + White Chestnut (accelerated repetition) + Cherry Plum (lack of control) + Holly (sudden outbreak).

In his lecture, Antonio Paramio explained his reasons for choosing the remedies in the kennel cough formula.

Beech to deal with irritative cough and intolerance to infectious agents.

Centaury to stop the spread of the infection and to boost the animal's immune system. Efficient energy supply to break the animal's pattern of submission to the infectious agents.

Cherry Plum because the disease's outbreak spreads quickly and uncontrollably. Cough out of control.

Crab Apple to cleanse the respiratory airways eliminating mucus and fluids.

Holly for its close association with the bile and also because the crises manifest as sudden outbreaks (eruptions).

Vervain to treat the inflammation of the respiratory airways and for excessive swelling (the infection tends to get worse).

White Chestnut for the accelerated repetition of coughing in each crisis.

When a Bach Flower treatment is to be applied to a large group of animals (animal shelters, farms, zoos, etc.) that share a disease or a common behaviour, the formula is prepared in a different way (see 'Concentrate formula', p.30).

For kennel cough, it is also advisable to treat puppies, older dogs and those dogs initially affected by the disease with an oral formula prepared in the standard way (see 'Preparation of a remedy for oral application', p.21).

Results from an experiment on kennel cough at the Amics dels Animals de la Noguera shelter

The dogs affected by the disease outbreak were treated with doxycycline and a Bach Flower oral formula (4 drops, two times per day). Two drops of the concentrate formula per litre of water were poured in each trough. Each time the troughs were refilled the drops of the concentrate formula were also added.

The symptoms of the animals responsible for the disease outbreak disappeared after four days of treatment with doxycycline and Bach Flower Remedies. The administration of combined treatment for two days to the first animals that showed symptoms of infection was enough to eliminate their cough. Animals that entered the shelter while the treatment was being administered, and therefore drank from the troughs with Bach Flower Remedies, were not infected.

Conclusions

The Bach Flower treatment showed great efficacy at a preventive level as animals that entered the shelter during the disease outbreak were not infected. The healing period was also shortened by combining drug therapy with Flower Remedies – it normally takes 10 to 12 days of treatment with doxycycline for the symptoms to disappear and for the animal to be cured, but the symptoms disappeared in only four days when the animals were treated with a combination of drug therapy and Bach Flower Remedies.

Colds due to low winter temperatures

Colds are more common in places where there are many animals and the weather is cold. It is important to resolve this issue for cats because when they catch a cold they lose their sense of smell and find it more difficult to recognize food. This is not a problem for a cat that lives in a house and has a family that controls the amount of food it eats. However, cats that live in large areas, as in the case of animal shelters, can become malnourished if they lose their sense of smell.

A preventive treatment is recommended, with the remedies listed below, and should start one month prior to the winter period and continue until the weather is milder (see 'Concentrate formula', p.30).

> Centaury (weakness, submission) + Crab Apple (cleanse) + Gorse (submission) + Olive (energy input) + Walnut (adaptation).

In any physical situation where the immune system is involved, the use of Gorse is a must. It deals with patterns of submission, boosting the animal's immune system. Centaury will also strengthen its immune system by enhancing resistance to infectious agents. Olive will provide extra energy input to address any possible invasion of pathogenic microorganisms. Walnut will help the animal to adapt better to adverse weather conditions. Finally, as always, Crab Apple will cleanse the animal's physical body in case of infection.

Results from an experiment on the preventive treatment of colds at the Amics dels Animals de la Noguera shelter

Due to the limited available volunteer staff, the animal shelter decided to carry out the study only in the feline population since cats are much more likely to catch colds than dogs. Moreover, when cats get sick they often have more complications (excessive mucus, loss of sense of smell and loss of the instinct to seek food).

The preventive treatment was carried out during the four coldest months of the winter season. Only one third of the feline community caught a cold, whereas the infectious outbreak the previous year when there was no Bach Flower treatment had affected all of the cats.

9

USEFUL FORMULAS

Abscesses

Also for lumps, fistulas, pimples, nodules, etc. Cream prepared with a neutral base cream or Aloe Vera gel.

> Crab Apple (cleanse) + Elm (pain sensitive to touch) + Vervain (inflammation) + Vine (if there is fluid in its interior, e.g. pus).

Minimum two applications per day.

Colds

> Centaury (weakness, submission) + Crab Apple (cleanse) + Gorse (submission) + Olive (energy input) + Walnut (adaptation).

4 drops, four times per day. (See Chapter 8, p.229).

Conjunctivitis

Eye-drops made with sterile saline solution.

> Beech (irritation) + Crab Apple (cleanse) + Vervain (inflammation).

2 drops in each affected eye, minimum two times per day.

Epilepsy

How Bach Flowers can help in the process of the disease

Idiopathic epilepsy is the most common cause of seizures in dogs. Although it may appear sporadically in almost all breeds and also in crossbred dogs, it is particularly frequent in certain pure breeds where the disease is considered hereditary, as in the case of the German shepherd, beagle, teckel, St Bernard and cocker spaniel. It is not as common in cats.

A typical epileptic seizure starts with sudden loss of consciousness and generalized stiffness, followed by erratic movements of head and limbs, urination and salivation. Sometimes seizures are milder: there is no loss of consciousness but there is an alteration of the state of mind, incoordination and more discreet body movements. The crises usually last between one and three minutes, and the recovery phase, of a variable duration, usually includes disorientation or other neurological signs.

REMEDIES ADMINISTERED ORALLY

(Refer to 'Preparation of a remedy for oral application', p.21.)

- Rock Rose: To treat diseases that occur sporadically, for no apparent reason. As Dr Bach (Bach 1936) said in his definition of Rock Rose:

  The remedy of emergency for cases where there even appears no hope. In accident or sudden illness, or when the patient is very frightened or terrified, or if the condition is serious enough to cause great fear to those around. If the patient is not conscious the lips may be moistened with the remedy.

- Cherry Plum: Compulsive episodes.

- Clematis: The typical crisis is characterized by starting with a sudden loss of consciousness.

- Vervain: Compulsive muscular hyperactivity.

- Beech: General stiffness.

- Scleranthus: Cyclicity of the disease.

- Chestnut Bud: Repetition of the crises and lack of coordination during the loss of consciousness.

Females in heat

Rescue Remedy + Beech (irritability) + Holly (hypersensitivity in this period) + Scleranthus (hormonal stabilizer) + Walnut (adaptation).

4 drops, four to six or more times per day depending on the animal to be treated.

Firework celebrations

Rock Rose (panic) + Star of Bethlehem (trauma, shock) + Sweet Chestnut (extreme distress) + Rescue Remedy (emergency).

If the animal has high stress levels add Vervain (overexcitement) and/or White Chestnut (repetition) to its formula. For dosage and preventive treatment, see Section 5.11.1, p.125.

Infection and abscess of the anal glands

Cream made with a neutral base cream or Aloe Vera gel.

Crab Apple (cleanse) + Star of Bethlehem (cicatrizant, promotes the healing of a wound) + Vervain (inflammation) + Walnut (cut, blood-clotter).

If the abscess does not drain out also add Vine (liquid causing pressure).

Minimum two applications per day.

Inflammation and infection of the third eyelid

Eye-drops prepared with sterile saline solution.

> Beech (irritation) + Crab Apple (cleanse) + Vervain (inflammation).

If in one week the swelling of the gland does not subside, add Vine (liquid causing pressure).

2 drops in each affected eye, minimum two times per day.

Learning process

> Cerato (trust and self-confidence) + Clematis (improves attention) + Chestnut Bud (assimilation, learning process) + Larch (disability) + Rock Water (resistance to change) + Walnut (adaptation).

4 drops, four times per day.

Mastitis

Cream made with a neutral base cream or Aloe Vera gel.

> Beech (irritation) + Crab Apple (cleanse) + Holly (rash) + Star of Bethlehem (trauma) + Vervain (inflammation) + Chicory (congestion and retention).

Minimum two applications per day.

Otitis

Prepared with sterile saline solution.

> Crab Apple (cleanse) + Elm (overwhelming pain) + Vervain (inflammation) + Vine (liquid causing pressure).

Formula from Orozco (2003).
2 drops inside the affected ear, minimum two times per day.

Skin allergy

For allergy to the contents of the anti-parasite pipettes, to fleas or other parasites, to plants, etc. cream made with a neutral base cream or Aloe Vera gel.

> Agrimony (unbearable itching) + Beech (irritation) + Crab Apple (cleanse) + Vervain (inflammation).

Minimum two applications per day.

Traumatisms

Being run over by a car, a fall, a bone fracture, a contusion, etc. Cream made with a neutral base cream or Aloe Vera gel.

> Elm (overwhelmed due to overload of any type) + Hornbeam (occasional weakness of the area to be treated) + Star of Bethlehem (traumatism) + Larch (if there is inability to move the affected part) + Vervain (if there is inflammation).

Minimum two applications per day.

Travel sickness (car journeys)

> Cherry Plum (lack of control) + Scleranthus (instability) + Walnut (adaptation) + Rescue Remedy (emergency).

If the animal has to travel by airplane inside a cage, add the following remedies to the above formula:

> Rock Rose (panic) + Sweet Chestnut (anxiety/anguish).

4 drops, four times per day. Start treatment one week before the trip. For short journeys by car, simply start treatment the day before (see Section 5.11.6, p.129).

Visits to the veterinarian pre- and postoperation

> Rescue Remedy (emergency) + Rock Rose (panic) + Star of Bethlehem (trauma) + Sweet Chestnut (extreme distress) + Olive (exhaustion due to stress, energy input).

For dosage, see Section 5.11.5, p.128.

Wounds

Formula made with still mineral water and Flower Remedies. Soak a sterile gauze with a few drops of the formula and apply to the wound for a few seconds.

> Crab Apple (cleanse) + Star of Bethlehem (cicatrizant, promotes the healing of a wound) + Vervain (inflammation) + Walnut (cut, blood-clotter) + Rescue Remedy (emergency).

Minimum two applications per day.

10

NEUTERING

Questions and Answers
(by the Altarriba Foundation)

Having an animal sterilized is one of the decisions that indicates the responsibility you have assumed. This chapter is worth reading because there are so many myths and urban legends surrounding this issue.

What is sterilization?

Sterilization is a surgical procedure that prevents the animal from reproducing. It can be carried out in males (vasectomy) and females (tubal ligation). In both cases the sexual organs and sexual behaviour remain intact as there is no modification of the hormonal processes. Females continue to be in heat.

What is neutering?

Neutering is the surgical removal of the sexual organs. Males: testes (castration), females: ovaries (ovariectomy: OV), or ovaries and uterus (ovariohysterectomy: OVH). Hormonal processes disappear and the animal's character remains unchanged (aggressiveness due to sexual dominance can eventually disappear in males). Females are never in heat.

What is recommended?

Undoubtedly, neutering is recommended for the reasons detailed in this chapter. These reasons are not just protectionist (reducing overpopulation and abandonments), but also apply to the direct wellbeing of the animal in question.

Why do you want to prevent the animal from enjoying its sexual life?

Animals do not experience sexuality as humans do because they have not taken the emotional step that this implies. For an animal, sex is only the physical process of reproduction. If eating and drinking is the guarantee of individual survival, sex is the guarantee of the species' continuity. In humans sex is an end in itself but in the rest of the animal world its only purpose is to conceive offspring, therefore the concept of enjoyment cannot be taken into consideration.

The clearest evidence of this is that female animals only accept being mounted when they are in heat, that is, when there is a hormonal demand. When the female animal is not in heat, she will refuse to have sex and may even reject males in a very aggressive manner. This shows how, for female animals, sex is a hormonal necessity and is not related to pleasure. Likewise, male animals only have the impulse to mount when they receive chemical information from a female in heat.

Will you be sad at having your animal neutered?

You can love your pet immensely, but do not put it into a human context where it does not belong. We have noted that when the vet suggests castration to a male owner, the latter tends to 'protect himself' as if the recommendation were for him. This reaction is understandable but very amusing. Castration, like vaccination, is in the animal's best interest; if owners do not feel scandalized when the vet suggests vaccination and are not saddened to have their pets undergo injections, the same should apply to castration.

Will my pet put on weight?

If an animal is overfed it will put on weight regardless of whether it has been neutered or not. In either case you must be very careful to control its diet and to provide adequate physical exercise for it to stay healthy. If the animal is going to be operated on and has a tendency to put on weight, the vet will give you specific instructions to avoid this; you just have to follow them to the letter.

Will it change its character?

Only hormone-associated behaviours change as a direct consequence of neutering, for example territoriality and facing-off with other animals in males. In many cases, animals have remarkable behavioural changes when they notice their owners treat them differently. This is the case when an owner becomes much more protective because he feels saddened to have neutered the animal and allows it to do things he would not have allowed previously.

Is it good for a female to breed at least once?

No. This is a myth. We are talking about hormonal and chemical processes here. If they are neutered they have no drive to reproduce, and will therefore have no psychological pregnancies, stress or seasonal anxiety. The maternal instinct in females disappears entirely (plus all its associated problems) with the OVH.

Do veterinarians suggest neutering in order to make money?

Vets are qualified professionals who have chosen animal health as their career (they have trained for many years). They suggest neutering because it is their obligation to look after the animal's interests. This applies to the animal in question and its possible future offspring; they recommend sterilization or neutering as they are convinced that the animal will be better off (e.g. to avoid a future pyometra and sudden death in the female).

What are the health benefits?

Neutering will prevent psychological pregnancies, pyometra and some breast tumours in females. In males it will prevent (amongst other conditions) testicular tumours, perineal hernias, hepatoid gland tumours, perineal gland tumours, prostate tumours and cysts, which according to veterinary statistics are currently on the increase.

Is it expensive?

The costs of surgery depend on the animal's characteristics – sex, size, age, etc. – and rates are generally recommended by each College of Veterinary Surgeons. Whatever the price it will be a bargain compared to the total cost of caring for the female during the two months of pregnancy and two months caring for the puppies (which means costly medication, special foods, possible complications, etc.). Therefore, if you are money conscious and take into consideration the fact that you will be saving money by avoiding your pet's future health problems, you will no doubt be interested in neutering your pet.

Will neutering your pet economically benefit pet shops and breeders?

The pet trade is nowadays governed by law and subject to compliance with the regulations in this regard, including licences, taxes, etc. We do not like this trade, but at present it is legal although we are working to end it. Nevertheless, once our point of view has been made clear it should be pointed out that almost 90 per cent of abandoned animals were not born with legal breeders or stores: they came from normal homes ('How wonderful to have a litter from my pet,' 'The neighbours have asked for a puppy from my pet,' 'I have found owners for all of them,' 'I will breed at home in order to sell the offspring for cash below market price,' 'There was a mistake and my dog has become pregnant,' 'I use the puppies to beg and when they grow up I will kill them and replace them with new puppies,' etc.).

Remember that the sterilization and neutering of animals will not create a greater volume of business for shops and breeders but will avoid a greater volume of adoptions in kennels and shelters.

Are we entitled to deprive animals of what nature has given them?

It depends, because avoiding an entire three-day-old litter being thrown into a river in a bag or crushed in a garbage truck is more important than a female's right to breed. To consider whether we have that right or not, we must first fulfil our obligations.

On the other hand, nature has given humans the same reproductive capability, but they exercise their right to not reproduce by using abundant contraceptive methods. At present, if it can be avoided, no woman has as many children as fertile years (one per year) and no man demands that from her. Nature and/or God have dictated the same laws for everyone. Do not use the argument that a female animal has the right to breed, that is, do not demand from others what you reject for yourself. Let's not be hypocritical.

My animal is purebred

In this case, please use another argument: your puppy might be one of those pedigree puppies that will end up on the street, in a kennel or in a shelter. In addition, the following issues affect purebreds: the owner gets rid of them when they grow old (as they must pay them more attention and time), sick (they must pay more for health care) or both. Do you know how many purebred animals end up living a hellish life? Do you know how many of them arrive old, blind, with cancer, and so on, at the animal shelters? However, mind you, they are 'very pure'. Some cases we've heard of recently include a 13-year-old dog, almost paralyzed, its mouth devastated by infections. However, it had an incredible pedigree, being son and grandson of champions. The owners got rid of it when it was no longer able to 'pose' with its pedigree. We also received a 19-year-old poodle (Trufita) weighing 1.3 kg at the shelter. She had been abandoned in a dumpster, was blind and had two tumours the size of tennis balls, one in each groin. She was very pure, a real 'toy', and must have cost the owners a fortune.

Will it be less of a guard dog?

The animal's personality does not depend as much on sexual hormones as it does on its genetic heritage and environment. Hence its tendency to protect its loved ones (you, the owner) will not be affected. If you really want to have security you should buy an alarm instead of a dog.

I really want to be present at a birth

Attending a birth is certainly a wonderful experience, and in the case of children it also teaches them to respect and care for animals. A newborn baby animal is fragile and beautiful, and awakens compassion in general (even though there are those who will throw them into the river in a sack).

If you want to experience a birth at home and allow your children to learn to respect the life of others you do not need your dog or cat to be pregnant. You can call the nearest animal shelter and you will undoubtedly be able to foster a female in need of care and about to give birth. You can take her home, take care of her, and enjoy two or three months taking care of the baby animals until they can be adopted. It will be a two-fold beautiful experience: the life that begins before your eyes and your generosity towards mistreated animals. The animal shelter will not know how to thank you.

I want to have offspring from my pet

Forget about any of your animal's puppies being its photocopy. It is understandable that you want to prolong the existence of your beloved animal as much as possible, even forever if you could. It is true that for you there will not be another one like it. That is the reason why you should not try to replace it specifically with another one of its own blood. Let this animal be special and unique and when it is gone, take the time you need before you share your life with another animal. Your new pet will also be special and will not come to replace the previous one but to continue sharing the happiness that has been interrupted momentarily by pain.

I will be responsible for the offspring

Nobody doubts it, but listen closely: you will have a litter that you will give to people close to you whom you trust. Each one of those people has the same right as you to enjoy the same enthusiasm and may want to continue breeding.

Look at Table 10.1 and think about it. Suppose that a female has only two litters in her life (cat 6 + 6, dog 4 + 4), and suppose that half of her offspring are females that breed in the same proportion (twice in their lives), and 100 per cent of the females survive.

Table 10.1 The number of offspring of one female cat and one female dog over five generations

	1 Cat	1 Dog
1st generation	12	8
2nd generation	84	40
3rd generation	588	200
4th generation	4,116	1,000
5th generation	28,812	5,000

After five generations, one cat and one dog give rise to a total amount of 33,812 animals, of which almost certainly 90 per cent (30,430) will die in kennels, streets, dogfights, poisoned, maimed, etc. This result will be the responsibility of the owner of the original animal.

Can you guarantee that you will be responsible for those thousands of animals that are the result of your first dream? Doesn't it worry you that the offspring of your beloved animal, bearing its same blood, will have this future? If this is the case you should take responsiblity and prevent this from happening.

No one makes money if I have a litter

Wrong. Based on the figures above, the following groups and individuals can make a lot of money from the offspring of your beloved animal.

- Companies (almost always dedicated to pest control, rat poisons, etc.) that manage municipal kennels and charge a certain fee per death (we will spare you from knowing how the grandchildren of your pets die in these centres).

- Dog-fight mafias that use the abandoned animals in order to 'train' their 'champions'.

- Textile trade mafias who make money from the animals' skin (coat cuffs and collars, baby booties, stuffed animal toys, etc.).

- Individuals who collect abandoned puppies in order to sell and/or breed them (if they find them 'cute').

- People who use abandoned animals in order to beg and keep them on the street, drugged and experiencing terrible weather conditions so they provoke more compassion.

References

Bach, E. (1931) *Heal Thyself*. London: The CW Daniel Company Ltd.

Bach, E. (1934) *The Twelve Healers and the Seven Helpers*. London: The CW Daniel Company Ltd.

Bach, E. (1936) *The Twelve Healers and Other Remedies*. London: The CW Daniel Company Ltd.

Noriega, P. (2006) 'Construyendo Puentes entre la Medicina Tradicional China y las Flores de Bach' (Building Bridges between Chinese Traditional Medicine and Bach Flowers). Workshop presented by SEDIBAC, 11 May, Barcelona.

Orozco, R. (2003) *Flores de Bach: Manual de Aplicaciones Locales*. Barcelona: Ed. Indigo.

Orozco, R. (2007) 'Bach Flowers and their application to animals: Ten years of research in animal shelters, working methods and action guidelines.' Talk presented at SEBIDAC, 5 May 2007, Barcelona.

Paramio, A. (2009) 'Kennel cough.' Presentation at SEDIBAC-SEFLOR Congress, Barcelona, 23 May 2009.

Rugaas, T. (1997) *On Talking Terms with Dogs: Calming Signals*. Washington: Dogwise Publishing.

Weeks, N. (1940) *The Medical Discoveries of Edward Bach, Physician*. London: The CW Daniel Company Ltd.

Further Reading

Barnard, J. and Barnard, M. (1996) *The Healing Herbs of Edward Bach: An Illustrated Guide to the Flower Remedies*. London: Ashgrove Publishing Ltd.

Bekoff, M. (2007) *The Emotional Lives of Animals: A Leading Scientist Explores Animal Joy, Sorrow, and Empathy and Why They Matter*. Novato, CA: New World Library.

Chancellor, P. (1971) *Illustrated Handbook of the Bach Flowers Remedies*. London: The CW Daniel Company Ltd.

Donaldson, J. (2005) *Culture Clash*. Berkeley, CA: James & Kenneth Publishers.

Eaton, B. (2007) *Dominance: Fact of Fiction?* Wenatchee, WA: Dogwise Publishing.

Grandin, T. (2005) *Animals in Translation: Using the Mysteries of Autism to Decode Animal Behavior*. New York: Scribner.

Masson, J.M. (1998) *Dogs Never Lie about Love: Reflections on the Emotional World of Dogs*. CA: Three Rivers Press.

McConnell, P.B. (2002) *The Other End of the Leash*. New York: Ballantine Books.

O'Heare, J. (2003) *Canine Neuropsychology*. Ottawa: Dogpsych.

O'Heare, J. (2007) *Aggressive Behavior in Dogs: A Comprehensive Technical Manual for Professionals*. Ottawa: DogPsych Publishing.

Rugaas, T. (2005) *My Dog Pulls. What Do I Do?* Wenatchee, WA: Dogwise Publishing.

Scheffer, M. (1988) *Bach Flower Therapy: Theory and Practice*. Rochester, VT: Healing Arts Press.

SEDIBAC (2001–2006) *Journals 29–44*. Barcelona. Available at www.sedibac.org/boletin.htm, accessed on 8 June 2011, or from info@sedibac.org.

SEDIBAC (2007–2009) *Journals 45–51*. Barcelona. Available at www.sedibac.org/boletin.htm, accessed on 8 June 2011, or from info@sedibac.org.

Sondermann, C. (2008) *Playtime for Your Dog: Keep Him Busy Throughout the Day*. Richmond: Cadmos Books.

Weeks, N. (1940) *The Medical Discoveries of Edward Bach, Physician*. London: The CW Daniel Company Ltd.

Index